ATLAS OF GRAY SCALE ULTRASONOGRAPHY

ATLAS OF GRAY SCALE ULTRASONOGRAPHY

KENNETH J. W. TAYLOR, B.Sc., M.D., Ph.D.

Associate Professor, Department of Diagnostic Radiology,
Yale University School of Medicine, New Haven, Connecticut

 CHURCHILL LIVINGSTONE
NEW YORK EDINBURGH AND LONDON 1978

CHURCHILL LIVINGSTONE
Medical Division of Longman Inc.

Distributed in the United Kingdom by Churchill Livingstone, 23
Ravelston Terrace, Edinburgh EH4 3TL, and by associated
companies, branches and representatives throughout the world.

First published 1978

ISBN 0 443 08001 1

7 6 5

Library of Congress Cataloging in Publication Data
Taylor, Kenneth J.W.   1939-
    Atlas of gray scale ultrasonography.

    Includes bibliographical references.
    1.   Diagnosis, Ultrasonic—Atlases.   I.   Title.
II.   Title: Gray scale ultrasonography.   [DNLM:
1.   Ultrasonics—Diagnostic use—Atlases.   WB17 T243a]
RC78.7.U4T39   616.07′54   77–12379

849   —   616.07544 ✓

Printed in USA

·Preface

This book is intended for all those who wish to know the current clinical applications of gray scale ultrasound in the diagnosis and management of their patients. It is intended for radiologists for whom ultrasound is a new modality and who wish to gain some insight into the basic principles underlying ultrasonic display and the indications for carrying out ultrasound examinations. To established radiologists, this book is intended as an introduction to the present wide clinical applications of gray scale ultrasound. To the resident, it is hoped that this book will provide sufficient background knowledge for the boards in radiology.

This book is also intended for referring physicians who need to know the potential of this new modality in the diagnosis of their patients' problems. Gray scale ultrasound is a very new technique which has only been commercially available since the middle of 1974, although the author's experience and some of the scans reproduced in this book were obtained early in 1973 from equipment built by David Carpenter from George Kossoff's laboratory in Sydney, Australia. Similar or even superior results can now be obtained on commercially available equipment, and scans obtained on both Picker and Searle equipment are included.

It is fortunate that this university center has personnel who have had extensive experience in ultrasound, some of whom have contributed to this book. Dr. Arthur Rosenfield has enthusiastically employed ultrasound at this institution as a complementary modality to genito-urinary radiology. He has contributed extensively to the original literature, and our results are summarized in the renal section of this book. Dr. Bruce Simonds, trained under Dr. George Leopold in San Diego, amassed a wealth of experience by establishing an ultrasound facility in Lausanne, Switzerland, and has contributed greatly to the ultrasonic investigation of the pancreas at this center. We thank Dr. John Hobbins, also of this medical center, for his comments on my chapters on obstetrics and gynecology.

The scans we have used in this book were carried out by the physicians and technologists in this ultrasound section of the Department of Radiology, as well as by the author at the Royal Marsden Hospital in England between 1973 and 1975. Special appreciation for their efforts and technical excellence go to Ms. Rosamund Silverman and Ms. Denise Moulton. These technologists have contributed to the technical sections on the estimation of biparietal diameter and on the scanning of the spleen, respectively. I would like to thank our other ultrasound technicians, Ms. Paula Jacobson and Ms. Lori May—and our students, Ms. Patty Doyle, Ms. Andrea Testa, Ms. Carol Talmont, and Ms. Linda Kostrubiak, who now produce the scans on which we make our day-to-day diagnoses.

My special thanks go to my wife, Caroline, who has not only borne with patience the gestational pains of this book, but has also taken time out from her busy life as a senior medical student to contribute the hundreds of illustrations which appear as line diagrams.

Finally, I would like to thank Ms. Ellen Green, Senior Editor, Ian Dick, Chief Designer, and the staff of Churchill Livingstone, who have worked with enthusiasm and skill to publish this book.

Yale University Medical School
New Haven, Connecticut
1977

Kenneth J.W. Taylor

Acknowledgments

We thank the editors and publishers of the journals listed below for permission to reproduce the following figures:

Figure	Source
4.7A 4.14	Taylor, K.J.W., Carpenter, D.A., Hill, C.R. and McCready, V. R.: Grey-scale ultrasound imaging. *Radiology*, **119**:415–423, 1976.
4.16	Taylor, K.J.W., Sullivan, D., Rosenfield, A.T. and Gottschalk, A.: Grey-scale ultrasound and isotope scanning: complementary techniques for imaging the liver. *American Journal of Roentgenology*, **128**:277–281, 1977.
4.17A 4.19 4.21 4.44 4.46	Rosenfield, A.T. and Taylor, K.J.W.: Grey-scale ultrasound in the imaging of urinary tract disease. *Yale Journal of Biology and Medicine*, **50**:335–353, 1977.
4.22 upper and lower	Taylor, K.J.W.: Grey-scale ultrasound imaging: diagnosis of metastatic secreting cystadenocarcinoma of the ovary. *British Journal of Radiology*, **48**:937–939, 1975.
4.24 11.16 13.3 8.33	Taylor, K.J.W. and McCready, V.R.: A clinical evaluation of grey-scale ultrasonography. *British Journal of Radiology*, **49**:244–252, 1976.
4.27	Gilby, E.D. and Taylor, K.J.W.: Ultrasound monitoring of hepatic metastases during chemotherapy. *British Medical Journal*, **15**:371–373, 1975.
4.39 4.42 4.47	Taylor, K.J.W., Sullivan, D., Rosenfield, A.T. and Gottschalk, A.: Grey-scale ultrasound and isotope scanning: complementary techniques for imaging the liver. *American Journal of Roentgenology*, **128**:277–281, 1977.
5.18	Taylor, K.J.W., Carpenter, D.A. and McCready, V.R.: Ultrasound and scintigraphy in the differential diagnosis of obstructive jaundice. *Journal of Clinical Ultrasound*, **2**:105–116, 1974.
7.8 10.28A	Taylor, K.J.W. and Carpenter, D.A.: Current applications of diagnostic ultrasound. *Guy's Hospital Reports*, **123**:27–41, 1974.
8.2C 8.29 8.32	Cooke, J.H., III, Rosenfield, A.T. and Taylor, K.J.W.: Ultrasonic demonstration of intrarenal anatomy. *American Journal of Roentgenology*, in press, 1977.

Figure	Source
8.5 8.6 8.10 8.13 8.26C 8.30 8.34 8.37	Rosenfield, A.T. and Taylor, K.J.W.: Grey-scale ultrasound in the imaging of urinary tract disease. *Yale Journal of Biology and Medicine*, **50**:335–354, 1977.
8.7 8.16 8.18 8.19 8.26B	Rosenfield, A.T. and Taylor, K.J.W.: Grey-scale nephrosonography: current status. *The Journal of Urology*, **117**:2–6, 1977.
8.8A	Rosenfield, A.T., Taylor, K.J.W., Siegel, N.J., Rosenfield, N.S. and Moulton, D.H.: Grey-scale ultrasound in congenital renal disorders. In: White, D. and Brown, R.E.: *Ultrasound in Medicine*. 3A. Clinical Aspects. Plenum Press, New York, 1977.
8.15	Teele, R.L., Rosenfield, A.T. and Freedman, G.S.: The anatomic splenic flexure: an ultrasonic renal impostor. *American Journal of Roentgenology*, **128**:115–120, 1977.
8.24	Bearman, S.B., Hine, P.L. and Sanders, R.C.: Multicystic kidney: a sonographic pattern. *Radiology*, **118**:685-688, 1976.
8.31	Rosenfield, A.T. and Taylor, K.J.W.: Obstructed uropathy in the transplanted kidney: evaluation by grey-scale sonography. *The Journal of Urology*, **116**:101–102, 1976.
8.33	Sanders, R.C.: Renal ultrasound. *Radiologic Clinics of North America*, **13**:417-434, 1975.
9.7 9.8 9.9	Taylor, K.J.W.: Ultrasonic investigation of inferior vena-caval obstruction. *British Journal of Radiology*, **48**:1024–1026, 1975.
13.3 13.5	Taylor, K.J.W. and McCready, V.R.: Nuclear medicine and endocrinology. *Proceedings of the Royal Society of Medicine*, **68**:381–384, 1975.
14.1 upper and lower	Taylor, K.J.W.: Use of ultrasound in opaque hemithorax. *British Journal of Radiology*, **47**:199–200, 1974.

We also thank Dr. Mort Glickman for permission to publish the arteriograms in this book, Dr. Alex Gottschalk for the isotope scans, and Dr. John Hobbins for Fig. 10.28C.

Contributors

Contributions

Arthur T. Rosenfield, M.D.
Bruce D. Simonds, M.D.
Daniel C. Sullivan, M.D.

Technical assistance

Denise Moulton, A.R.D.M.S.
Rosamund Silverman, B.S., A.R.D.M.S.

Illustrations

Caroline Taylor, B.Sc.

All contributors are from the Yale University School of
Medicine, Yale-New Haven Hospital, New Haven, Connecticut

Contents

1. Basic principles of diagnostic ultrasound

INTRODUCTION

For diagnostic purposes ultrasound may be used in several different ways including sonar, Doppler, and holography. For present purposes, this discussion is limited to sonar, which is the use of short-pulse echo techniques to display two dimensional sections through soft tissues. Although sonar has been used with success in many clinical applications since the middle 1950s, suddenly 20 years later there has been a surge of renewed interest in the modality and a vast increase in the number of applications for the technique. Marked improvements in technology have been responsible for these changes in the usefulness of this modality, and these modifications are summarized by the use of the term "gray scale ultrasonography," which has replaced the previous bistable techniques. Much of this improved technology was evolved by Kossoff and his co-workers of the Ultrasonic Institute in Sydney, Australia, who reported the clinical value of the technique in obstetrics, gynecology, breast, and thyroid (Kossoff, 1974a and b). A similar machine was evaluated in England which demonstrated the value of the technique when applied to the investigation of the hepatobiliary tract (Taylor, Carpenter, and McCready, 1973; Taylor and McCready, 1976; Taylor, Carpenter, McCready *et al.*, 1976). It became apparent that the adoption of gray scale techniques provided the ultrasonologist with much more information than he had hitherto available so that a new generation of high-quality gray scale instruments was introduced commercially in 1974. It is the widespread commercial availability of these improved machines that has led to the present exponential increase in the applications and clinical value of the technique (Leopold, 1975; Campbell and Wilkin, 1975; Carlsen and Filly, 1976; Filly and Carlsen, 1976).

The basic principles of diagnostic ultrasound are first reviewed.

BASIC PRINCIPLES

Frequencies employed

Although ultrasound refers to sound waves at frequencies in excess of those audible to the human ear or approximately 15 000 cycles per second (15 KHz), for medical diagnostic applications, frequencies in the 1 to 10 MHz range must be employed to obtain the required resolution. As with light, the obtainable resolution is dependent upon the wavelength, λ, which is related to the frequency, F, and the velocity, C, of an ultrasound beam as:

$$F \times \lambda = C \qquad \text{equation 1}$$

Thus, at a frequency of 1 MHz and a velocity of approximately 1500 Ms^{-1} in soft tissue, the wavelength is 1.5 mm.

It is apparent from equation 1 that the wavelength varies inversely with the frequency so that better resolution can be obtained by employing higher frequencies. However, tissue attenuation also increases almost linearly with frequency, and this limits the depth to which tissue may be imaged. Thus, in the examination of deeply placed organs, the frequency employed is a compromise between the highest frequency for optimal resolution but which still permits adequate penetration. In practice, this will be about 2.25 MHz for most large patients, 3 to 3.5 MHz for thin patients, and 5 MHz for superficial organs such as the thyroid, for newborns and for young children.

Production of ultrasound

Ultrasound beams at frequencies in the MHz range are generated by the piezoelectric effect. A property displayed by some naturally occurring crystals, such as quartz, is the development of an electrical potential across them when they are compressed (see Fig. 1.1A). The reverse phenomenon is used in the production of ultrasound and, for convenience, synthetic ceramics are used instead of quartz. One such transducer material is a barium titanate-lead zirconate ceramic (PZT-5 Brush-Clevite) in the form of a disc. An electrical potential is placed across the ceramic which responds by undergoing mechanical deformation. If a single electrical pulse of microseconds' duration is used to energize the transducer, a short series of compressions and rarefactions are transmitted into the adjacent medium, as shown schematically in Figure 1.1A.

An ultrasound transducer tends to ring like a bell for several cycles after being activated, and this effect is minimized by the choice of the material for the ceramic. The number of sound wave cycles emitted from a

1

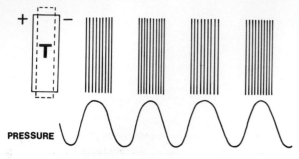

PRESSURE

Fig. 1.1A Schema to show production of continuous wave ultrasound by a transducer (T). A man-made ceramic is subjected to a potential difference across its face, and this causes it to undergo mechanical deformation (dotted lines). When the transducer is not subjected to a potential difference, it returns to its resting geometry, and this has produced a pressure wave followed by a rarefaction in the propagating medium. The rate at which the electrical pulses are delivered to the transducer dictates the frequency of the sound wave emitted. The lower schema shows a pressure wave which constitutes the sound wave.

transducer in response to a single energizing electrical pulse is known as the mechanical Q of the transducer. This is analogous to the ringing of a bell after being struck. For quartz, the mechanical Q is 1500 and such long pulses would preclude satisfactory axial resolution if used as a transducer material. In comparison, PZT-5 has a mechanical Q of 50 which is still too long for optimal resolution using short-pulse echo techniques. The pulse length is further decreased by heavily damping the back of the transducer, analogous to the short response from a bell in contact with an absorbing material. This combination of a suitable transducer material and heavy damping results in the emission of a

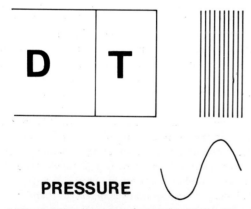

PRESSURE

Fig. 1.1B Schema to show the production of an idealized single sound wave. The transducer (T) is heavily damped by backing material (D) continuous with the back face of the transducer. This shortens the resulting pulse wave, like holding a bell to prevent after-ringing. This damping results in a very short train of pulses, represented ideally as a single sine wave.

very short pulse approximating 1 wavelength in duration (Fig. 1.1B).

After emission of such a short pulse of ultrasound, the transducer is used to receive the returned echoes and convert this reflected acoustic energy into signals which can be suitably amplified, processed, and displayed. The sonar mode of usage consists of approximately 1 microsecond emission for sound energy and 1000 microseconds (1 millisecond) for receiving. Thus, 1000 pulses may be emitted per second, and the transducer used to listen for echoes for 99.9 % of the time during the scanning process. A clear understanding of this is necessary to appreciate the safety of diagnostic ultrasound, which is largely due to the very short pulses of energy emitted compared with the time constants for any mechanical or physical reaction and the low average delivery of energy because the transducer functions as a passive receiver for 99.9 % of the time.

Intensity of ultrasound
The intensity of ultrasound is measured in $W\ cm^{-2}$. This is an absolute measurement of power which may be measured by the pressure exerted by the ultrasound beam. A pressure of 67 mg is produced by an ultrasonic intensity of $1\ W\ cm^{-2}$. The maximum intensity of the transmitted pulse in diagnostic ultrasound may be as high as $100\ W\ cm^{-2}$, although machines are seldom used at full power and peak intensities of around $1\ W\ cm^{-2}$ are more common. Since the equipment is passively receiving for 99.9 % of the time, the average power transmitted through tissues in diagnostic ultrasound is in the range of a few $mW\ cm^{-2}$. When considering the simple physics involved in the behavior of ultrasound, it is more convenient to use relative measurements of power, which is the decibel notation. This is a logarithmic notation so that variations of 1 dB imply a change by a factor of 10 in absolute power levels.

The reflection process
A short pulse of ultrasound, ideally a single sine wave cycle, travels through the transmitting medium at a velocity characteristic of that medium. On reaching an interface with a medium of different acoustic properties, the ultrasound beam may be reflected or refracted similar to the behavior of light at the junction of media of different refractive indices. The characteristic acoustic impedance of a medium is the equivalent acoustic property, and this is designated by Z, which is the product of C, the velocity of sound in that medium, and ρ, which is the density of that medium. Thus:

$$Z = \rho \times C \qquad \text{equation 2}$$

At an interface between media of different acoustic impedances, Z_1 and Z_2, a component of the sound wave energy will be reflected while most of the beam will be

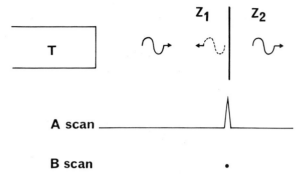

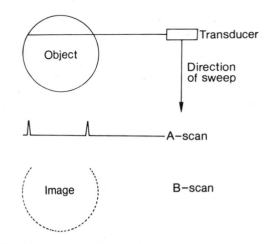

Fig. 1.2 Schema to show single sine wave emitted from the transducer face (T). This ultrasound pulse is transmitted through medium with an acoustic impedance of Z_1. On reaching the interface between media 1 and 2, the sound energy will behave like light and be partly reflected. If Z_1 and Z_2 are of similar magnitude, most of the sound wave energy will be propagated into the medium with an acoustic impedance of Z_2. The dotted pulse represents the small reflected component which is returned to the transducer. The interface between media 1 and 2 is represented on the oscilloscope tube in one of two ways. In the A-scan, the amplitude of the reflected component is modulated by the size of the deflection from the baseline so that a small spike is shown. The distance of the interface is computed by the time difference between the emission of the transmitted pulse and the receipt of the reflected component. Distance may be computed if the velocity is known. The B-scan presentation shows a brightness modulation of the interface which is represented by a single dot, the brightness of which is proportional to the amplitude of the reflected component.

Fig. 1.3 Schema to show the formation of a B-scan. The two sides of the object give rise to spikes on the A-scan and two dots on the B-scan. The two-dimensional aspects of the B-scan are generated by the movement of the transducer in a perpendicular plane to the object, as shown schematically.

transmitted into the second medium, as shown schematically in Figure 1.2.

The small echo emanating at this interface returns through medium 1 and impinges on the face of the transducer where it is changed into an electrical pulse and can be displayed. To locate the position of the interface at the correct distance from the transducer face, the velocity of sound in the transmitting medium must be assumed and the time can be measured for the ultrasound beam to reach and return from the interface. The correct position of the interface can then be recorded on the oscilloscope tube. The size of the echo can be registered in terms of the amplitude of the deflection of the spike from the baseline. This type of display is known as an A-mode, that is, *A*mplitude modulated.

An echo can also be *B*rightness modulated—the so-called B-mode. In this type of display, the larger the echo, the brighter the spot on the oscilloscope tube. A single echo will be represented as a single spot; but when the transducer is moved in a plane normal to the direction of the ultrasound beam, a two-dimensional image is generated providing the echoes are stored. This is shown schematically in Figure 1.3.

A B-scan is a two-dimensional scan in which the axes (XY coordinates) are spatial. A two-dimensional display can be formed in which the X axis is distance and the Y axis is time. This is achieved by a brightness modulated display of a single space dimension through an organ on a moving time base produced either by sweeping the cathode ray oscilloscope beam or by moving the recording paper. This is known as an M-mode tracing, as demonstrated in Figure 1.4. When a beam is passed across the left and right ventricles of the heart impinging on the mitral valve leaflets, the movements of these structures in time produces a characteristic recording. The M-mode records the movement of a single space dimension in time. A very considerable amount of information may be obtained about the heart and other rapidly moving structures from the examination of such a tracing. For example, the slope of the tracing of any moving structure is the velocity of motion. However, considerable expertise is required for interpretation and, in particular, to appreciate the orientation of the ultrasound beam through the heart during any particular part of the examination. The great advantage of real-time scanning (pp. 11–14) is the addition of the third dimension giving two spatial dimensions and their movements in time. This results in a cross section through the heart which is seen beating in real time. This permits easy spatial orientation of an M-mode recording since the various chambers and valves of the heart are easily identified in a cross-sectional display.

Resolution of ultrasound systems

As stated previously, the ultimate resolution of an ultrasound imaging system depends on the frequency

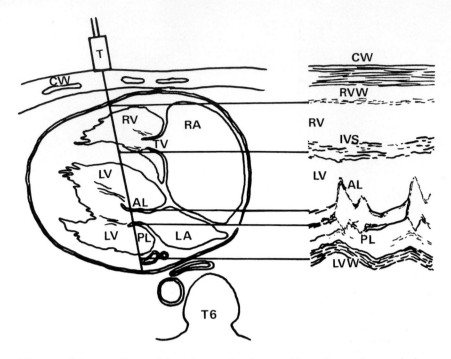

Fig. 1.4 Schema to show an M-mode scan. An ultrasound beam is passed across the heart in the anatomical position shown in the schema; the beam transects the right ventricle (RV), left ventricle (LV), and is incident upon both anterior (AL) and posterior (PL) mitral valve leaflets. The interventricular septum (IVS) can be seen between the ventricular cavities, the right ventricular wall (RVW) is seen anteriorly, and the chest wall (CW) intervenes between the heart and the transducer (T). The posterior left ventricular wall (LVW) is seen, as are the atria (RA and LA).

The tricuspid valve is designated TV. The line of ultrasonic data is brightness modulated and then the tracing is moved in time either mechanically or electrically, which results in a recording of the position of various heart structures as they move in time. Thus, an M-mode tracing is a two-dimensional recording—one spatial and one temporal—and the gradient of any line on the M-mode recording will be the velocity with which the structure moves, since it is the rate at which the structures are moving in time.

employed, which therefore must be as high as is consistent with the desired depth of penetration. However, at any given frequency other factors affect the resolution. Since B-scans are two-dimensional, factors affecting the resolution in each plane must be considered. The plane of the transducer may be called the X axis or the axial plane. The resolution on the Y axis at right angles to the axial plane is termed the lateral resolution.

Resolution in the axial plane
This is dependent on the brevity of the ultrasound pulse. The duration of any echo cannot be shorter than the duration of the original transmitted pulse. If the pulse length approaches a single wavelength (0.75 mm at 2 MHz), the echo will be of similar brevity resulting in an axial resolution of 0.75 mm. If multiple sound wave cycles are present in the pulse and the echo is consequently longer, poor axial resolution must result.

Hence the importance of employing very short pulses of ultrasound to interrogate tissues; and these are produced by the combination of appropriate transducer materials with low mechanical Q and heavy damping to prevent ringing.

Lateral resolution
The lateral resolution of a transducer depends upon the beam width and this varies with the distance from the transducer face and the size of the face compared with the wavelength. Four possible types of ultrasound transducer field profiles are shown in Figure 1.5A-D. When the transducer face is small compared with the wavelength, a rapidly divergent beam is produced (Fig. 1.5A). The sequel is apparent if two reflectors, *A* and *B*, are considered. Both reflectors are illuminated by the ultrasound beam and give rise to echoes which are spatially inseparable. Thus these two points cannot be discriminated. Brief consideration of any other two

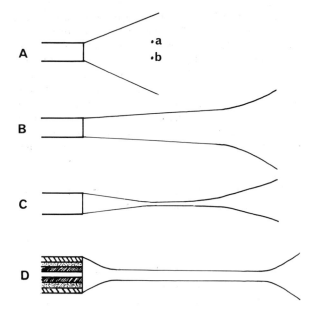

Fig. 1.5A A schematic field intensity profile of a transducer in which the wavelength is relatively large compared with the diameter of the transducer, producing a diverging beam. Note that two-point reflectors A and B within the beam will not be discriminated.
B A collimated beam is narrow near the transducer face but becomes wider with increasing distance from it.
C Medium-focused transducer. The beam is brought to a focus at a given distance from the transducer face and the beam width is greater both before and after this focal plane. The more strongly a beam is focused, the more limited the focal zone. For the purpose of surveying entire organs, a weakly or medium-focused transducer may be optimal to insure a long focal zone.
D Annular array of transducers in which a number of transducers are arranged concentrically, each with focal planes at different distances from the transducer. The use of each of these transducers insures a narrow beam path. Theoretically, these transducers should produce much superior resolution than the medium- and weakly focused transducers at present in clinical use. In practice to date, the improvements appear rather marginal.

points within the sound beam at the same distance from the transducer face leads to the realization that the lateral resolution of a transducer must be dependent upon the beam width. It should be appreciated that this consideration of beam width is simplified. There is an exponential decline in intensity away from the axis of the beam and, for descriptive purposes, the beam width is considered to include the ultrasound field, which is up to 20 dB less than the axial intensity. However, large reflectors outside this beam so defined may be confused with those within the conventional beam and this will cause artifacts due to "side lobes." Side lobes are therefore regions of ultrasound field intensity in which

large reflectors may give rise to significant echoes which are erroneously considered to have originated nearer the axis.

A less divergent ultrasound field can be produced with a larger transducer face, as shown in Figure 1.5B. Such a collimated beam is approximately parallel for a short distance from the transducer face but eventually shows wide diversion. This approach is used for high frequency transducers in the examination of superficial organs such as the thyroid. Such an arrangement is unsuited to the examination of deep tissues due to the spread of the ultrasound beam.

Figure 1.5C shows the usual transducer design for the examination of deep organs. The ultrasound beam is focused at a suitable depth by means of a plastic lens. Thus, for optimal resolution in different patients, not only must the optimal frequency be employed but a transducer used which focuses approximately at the depth of interest.

The ideal transducer would be approached by a design shown in Figure 1.5D in which the focal plane is extended to include the entire area of interest. This cannot be achieved by a single transducer, but this ideal may be approached by the future generation of annular arrays. These consist of a number of transducers concentrically arranged and each of which focuses at a different depth. Sequential use of each transducer effectively results in an extended focal plane, which is shown schematically in Figure 1.5D.

Tissue attenuation and TGC

Sound waves of any frequency are attenuated by passage through a transmitting medium. This attenuation is exponential and thus can easily be expressed in the logarithmic dB notation. Approximate values for the attenuation coefficient for soft tissues is 1.0 dB per cm per MHz (0.5 dB cm^{-1} MHz^{-1}) round trip for the transmitted and reflected paths. In normal soft tissues, most attenuation is due to absorption by protein macromolecules and a small fraction (about 20%) due to scatter and reflection.

Thus an ultrasound beam is rapidly attenuated by passage through tissue so that the incident intensity on a deeply seated reflector will be very small compared with the incident intensity on a superficially placed reflector. Furthermore, echoes originating from deeply placed reflectors will suffer attenuation during their return path to the transducer. Thus echoes from deeply seated structures will be small compared with echoes from less distant reflectors. However, selective amplification can be added to these small distant echoes to compensate for tissue attenuation, and this is referred to as time gain control (TGC). The TGC must approximate this tissue attenuation and this is 0.5 dB cm^{-1} MHz^{-1}. Therefore at a frequency of 3 MHz, 3.0 dB amplification is added to the signal for each cm of tissue depth. This means that echoes from a depth of 10 cm are selectively amplified 30 dB more than those originating near the skin surface. Since decibel scale is logarithmic, this represents an enormous power ratio which is required to compensate for tissue attenuation.

From the practical point of view of setting the required TGC, the objective is to achieve even-sized echoes throughout homogeneous tissues. This practical aspect is considered in detail in the section pertaining to liver (p. 15). It should be noted that tissue attenuation increases almost linearly with frequency so that adjustment of TGC is required when transducers of different frequencies are used.

Types of reflectors

Specular reflectors
By analogy to the behavior of light at a reflecting interface, two different types of physical reflecting processes may be considered. One of these is called a specular reflection and the other is back-scattered. A specular echo is analogous to the behavior of light when incident on a mirror. The reflecting beam is of large amplitude and the direction of the reflected beam is such that the angle of incidence equals the angle of reflection (Fig. 1.6A). Thus only when the beam approaches normal incidence to the reflecting interface does the path of the reflected component begin to coincide with the path of the incident beam (Fig. 1.6B). The amplitude of the returned echo is therefore highly dependent upon the orientation of the ultrasound beam

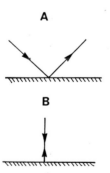

A

B

Fig. 1.6A A specular reflection is of large amplitude and arises at interfaces that are large compared with the wavelength. The reflection of energy is such that the angle of incidence equals the angle of reflection, so that the reflected component along the same path as the incident beam is highly dependent upon the angle of the beam to the reflecting interface.

B Specular echo at normal incidence to a reflector in which virtually all the sound energy incident on the reflector is returned along the same path. Thus, for specular reflectors, the amplitude of the reflected component is strongly dependent upon the angle of orientation.

to the reflecting interface. These echoes are very large in amplitude and therefore rather easy to display by relatively crude electronic techniques. It follows that the amplitude of the echoes depends predominantly upon the rather random orientation of the beam to reflecting interfaces. The older bistable machines largely displayed only these specular echoes of large amplitude which were markedly affected by angle of orientation. The information so obtained was limited to the display of contour information where the echoes were of large amplitude such as the fetal skull or at tissue/fluid interfaces.

For a specular echo the reflected component, R, of an ultrasound beam is given by the expression:

$$R = \frac{Z_1 - Z_2}{Z_1 + Z_2} \qquad \text{equation 3}$$

Where Z_1 and Z_2 are the acoustic impedance of medium 1 and 2 forming the interfaces. Substituting in equation 2,

$$R = \frac{\rho_1 C_1 - \rho_2 C_2}{\rho_1 C_1 + \rho_2 C_2} \qquad \text{equation 4}$$

Consideration of this formula allows us to predict the behavior of an ultrasound beam at a tissue/air interface. The density of air is negligible compared with the density of soft tissue, so that the reflected component approaches unity indicating virtually 100 % reflection at a tissue/air interface.

It may also be shown that the velocity, density and bulk modulus of a medium are related as:

$$c = \sqrt{\frac{B}{\rho}} \qquad \text{equation 5}$$

The bulk modulus of a medium is dependent upon the stiffness of the tissue or its rigidity. It is obvious that supporting tissues must be rigid and hence have a high bulk modulus. Supporting tissues in soft organs are due to collagen, elastin, and similar materials. These are referred to as the fibrous skeleton of soft organs.

Considering equation 3, there are only small differences in the published values for acoustic impedance between various soft tissues, and it is difficult to appreciate the origin of the rather large echoes which emanate from them. This difficulty is removed if equation 5 is substituted in equation 3. The reflected component then becomes:

$$R \simeq \frac{\sqrt{B_1} - \sqrt{B_2}}{\sqrt{B_1} + \sqrt{B_2}} \qquad \text{equation 6}$$

This relationship was pointed out by Fields and Dunn (1973), who noted that there are very large differences in the reported values for bulk moduli. In particular, the bulk moduli of collagen and similar supporting tissues are some 10 000 greater than the surrounding soft tissues. Thus, large differences do exist in the acoustic properties of soft organs and these could form the main site of echo formation.

If this proposal is true, then the display of liver, for example, is dependent upon the collagen supporting tissue in the blood vessels, biliary system and Glisson's capsule. An inflammatory reaction surrounding an abscess cavity would appear as a rim of high-level echoes. This has been clinically observed. In contrast, replacement of the normal anatomy by tumors or abscesses would appear as defects in the normal structure. This again is seen in the clinical situation. Thus, for present purposes, interpretation of gray scale ultrasound appearances should be based on the assumption that a major site of echo formation is collagen and similar supporting tissues.

Backscattered echoes
Another type of reflector produces a backscattered echo. This is shown schematically in Figure 1.6C. These

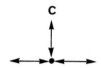

Fig. 1.6C Schema to show backscattered reflector in which the reflecting interface is small compared with the wavelength of the ultrasound beam. Such a reflector is omnidirectional and the amplitude of the reflected component is therefore independent of the angle of orientation.

reflectors are small compared with the wavelength and give rise to echoes of small amplitude. However, these echoes are returned in the same plane as the incident beam so that amplitudes of such echoes are largely independent of the angle of incidence. Highly important sequelae result from this independence of angle of incidence which have relevance to the interpretation of gray scale ultrasound scans and the technique for scanning. The properties of specular and backscattered echoes are summarized:

Specular echoes	*Backscattered echoes*
Large amplitude	Small amplitude
Amplitude highly dependent on angle of incidence	Amplitude independent of angle of incidence

It should be noted that it is necessary to approach normal incidence with a reflector before a reflection of large amplitude is obtained in the plane of the incident beam. Little of our visual perception of the surrounding

world is dependent upon specular echoes and most of our vision results from backscattered reflections. Specular reflectors constitute the highlights from a glass and similar reflecting surfaces. Yet the older bistable ultrasound machines were largely limited to the display of specular echoes; since these were few in number and highly directional in amplitude, complex scanning techniques were developed such as compounding to overcome these problems. Compounding consists of moving the transducer in small arcs to ensure, at least once, the ultrasound beam is at normal incidence to the reflecting interface. Since the amplitude of backscattered echoes is so independent of angle of orientation, there are obvious advantages to displaying these low-level echoes. One major feature of gray scale systems is the selective amplification of these low-level echoes, their retention and display.

Gray scale systems
Gray scale ultrasonography is characterized by two major improvements on the bistable systems previously employed: enhanced resolution and signal-to-noise ratio. Improved resolution is largely due to focused and collimated transducers, but the enhanced signal-to-noise ratio is fundamental to the new technology. The low-level echoes which originate from within soft tissues are amplified and displayed. This permits visualization of the fine internal consistency of soft tissues and the recognition of abnormal patterns which are characteristic of diffuse pathology. Small space-occupying lesions are best detected as defects in this normal anatomy, hence the importance of amplifying and displaying these low-level echoes.

The degree of amplification that is required for visualization of such fine structure presents distinct physical and engineering problems. The total range of echoes from tissue is about 100 dB. This vast range of intensity amplitudes is the difference between the smallest echo we wish to display and the largest, specular echo from the greatest discontinuity of acoustic impedance found in tissues. However, this large range is partly due to tissue attenuation, so that addition of TGC in the first stage of signal processing reduces the range of echoes to about 60 dB. This still greatly surpasses the dynamic range of the cathode ray oscilloscope tube (about 15 dB) and even TV systems (about 20 dB).

In the consideration of the types of reflectors within tissue (p. 6) it was noted that the largest echoes are specular in nature and their absolute amplitude is highly dependent upon the angle of orientation of the beam to the reflector. It seems unlikely that there is much useful clinical information in such random data so that, if the dynamic range of the display system is insufficient to linearly represent the whole range of echoes from tissues, then the smaller echoes must be retained and

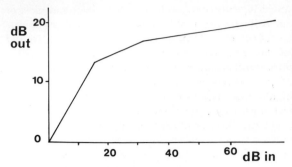

Fig. 1.7 Schema to show compression amplification principle in which a range of 60 dB is compressed into the limited dynamic range of the oscilloscope tube or television tube. Note the linear amplification of the lower level echoes while the larger echoes are increasingly compressed. It should be noted that small differences in the amplitude of echoes will be maintained only when the echoes are small. Excessive amplification of these echoes will bring them into the compression part of the curve, which minimizes the differences between them. In this way excessive gain can cause metastases in the liver to appear like normal tissue.

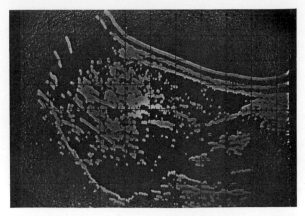

Fig. 1.8A Bistable B-mode ultrasonogram through liver and right kidney. Notice all echoes are shown at the same intensity, and any small echoes below the threshold level, which can be adjusted, are lost from the scan.

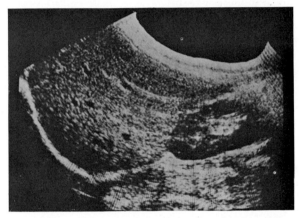

Fig. 1.8B Gray scale B-mode ultrasonogram through right lobe of the liver and kidney showing marked improvement in resolution and display of tissue consistency when echoes of various amplitudes are displayed in different shades of gray.

displayed at the cost of the larger, orientation-dependent specular echoes. This type of signal processing, which is known as compression amplification, is shown schematically in Figure 1.7. Given an input range of 60 dB, the low-level backscattered echoes are preferentially amplified. Medium- to high-level echoes are increasingly compressed, but this is clinically unimportant since differences in their amplitudes are so largely dependent upon angle of incidence.

In contrast, the amplitude of the low-level, backscattered echoes is independent of the orientation and is largely dependent upon the consistency of tissue and, in particular, on the collagen content. This does have clinical relevance because of the importance of fibrosis in many pathological processes. For example, diffuse intrahepatic fibrosis is characteristic of cirrhosis and it can be shown by A-scan analysis that significantly larger echoes emanate from the cirrhotic liver than the normal one. More localized fibrosis may be seen surrounding or in response to some tumors.

The differences between the gray scale display and the older bistable scans are demonstrated in Figure 1.8A and B. Fine resolution is apparent in the tissue consistency, and the limits of this fine structure define the organ contour. The bistable scan, in contrast, displays only the contour information and the low-level information on tissue consistency is lost either in the signal processing or in the display system. This type of scan was called bistable because of the all or none nature of the recording system. All echoes above a given intensity are registered at the same brightness, while lower-level echoes are below the threshold and hence not registered. In contrast, the gray scale display uses various shades of gray to represent echoes of different amplitudes. However, for adequate gray scale display, the low-level echoes must be selectively amplified. By analogy to light, the gray scale scan is directly similar to our visual perception, which is highly dependent on backscattered nonspecular reflections. The angular dependent specular echoes, which appear as "glare" or "highlights" in our visual perception, are not linearly amplified in the ultrasound signal processing and therefore do not saturate the display system.

Scanning techniques in gray scale ultrasonography

Scanning techniques that are widely used in clinical practice are still, in many instances, those necessitated predominantly by the old bistable technology. Echoes arising from major organ interfaces such as the fetal skull are predominantly specular and therefore are seen most efficiently when the ultrasound beam is at normal incidence to the reflector. It was this concept that gave rise to the technique of "compound scanning" in which the transducer was moved in small arcs to find the maximum echo when the beam was at normal incidence (Donald, McVicar, and Brown, 1958). Compound scanning is no longer a necessity to display the fine structure of tissues when the backscattered echoes have no such simple relationship to orientation and appear more nearly omnidirectional.

For complete transverse sections of the body, compound scanning is necessary and can be used to produce predominantly contour information. This may be very useful in certain clinical applications such as radiotherapy planning. Such techniques will, however, lead to severe degradation of resolution for the following simple physical reasons:

1. In compound scanning techniques, the ultrasound beam is incident upon the same reflector on many occasions from different angles of incidence in an attempt to maximize the returned echoes. In the upper abdomen where there are highly significant respiratory movements and cardiac pulsations, each point reflector will be written many times throughout its oscillatory excursion unless the imaging process is instantaneous. For manual scanning techniques, the ultrasound imaging process is not instantaneous so that biological movements will significantly degrade the attainable resolution.
2. When an echo is received from a distance from the transducer face, that distance is computed from the time of arrival of that pulse assuming a constant velocity of sound in tissue. In the clinical situation,

tissue is not homogeneous and velocities of sound in soft tissues do vary significantly. Thus the computation of the XY coordinates involved in the B-scan geometry is based on assumed velocities, and this again will result in degradation of resolution when a single point reflector is registered from a number of different positions.
3. The mechanical requirements for compounding are stringent in that a completely rigid arm is essential, but in clinical practice many mechanical arms show a considerable degree of slack.

The alternative to compound scanning is the use of linear, sector or single pass scans in which each element of tissue volume is interrogated once only so that subsequent movement of the tissue following registration and inaccuracies in sound velocity assumptions leads to only minimum distortion of the image and does not blur detail by repeated registrations. Thus, from the simple physical considerations enumerated here, compound scanning can be abandoned in most gray scale scans except where the information required is purely contour in nature. The advantage of using a single pass technique is greatly enhanced resolution. Scanning techniques in relation to individual organs are considered in the appropriate chapter, but the advantage of single pass techniques is shown in Figure 1.9, which shows a single pass across the upper abdomen transversely demonstrating the smaller branches of the celiac artery.

Recording systems

Static images

When considering permanent or hard copy recording systems, one must consider the quality of the image, the cost of hard copy, the ability to check the adequacy of the

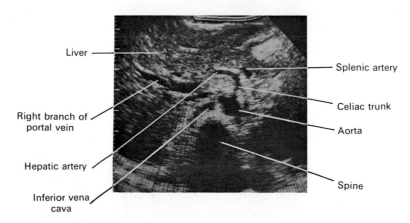

Liver

Splenic artery

Celiac trunk

Right branch of portal vein

Aorta

Hepatic artery

Inferior vena cava

Spine

Fig. 1.9 Transverse scan across the abdomen using single pass technique to show upper abdominal vascular anatomy.

record before the patient leaves the department, and the ease of archival storage and retrieval. No ideal system has yet become apparent for either ultrasound or computerized tomography. The most widely used system for both modalities is the static photography of a TV screen using Polaroid film. The major advantage of this system is the immediate availability of the record, which can be checked before any further scans of the patient are carried out and certainly before the patient leaves the department. Polaroid film is, however, extremely expensive and in many large centers this now results in expenditures exceeding $24,000 per annum. The results are technically adequate if the scan converter is optimally adjusted, but the photographic process tends to add a contrast to the original image; to optimize the result, it is necessary to allow for this increased contrast by adjustment of the photographed screen.

Largely because of the high price of Polaroid film, celluloid film has been increasingly used either in 35 mm, 70 mm, 90 mm or 110 mm format. A number of cameras are available for such photography and one great advantage is that the celluloid film is much less dependent upon the precise adjustment of the contrast and intensity levels. Such film is also very considerably less expensive than Polaroid. The major disadvantage devolves from the inability to immediately check the film and, when necessary, to make small adjustments to optimize photography. In a busy diagnostic unit, it is essential to ensure that such recordings are optimal and diagnostically adequate before the patient leaves the department. The vast majority of ultrasound services are physically located in the Radiology Department where an X-o-mat developer is usually in close proximity, and this results in the increasing use of X-ray film for diagnostic ultrasound recording.

X-ray film is used in a multiformat camera, resulting in a number of images, one, four or nine on a half-plate X-ray film (Fig. 1.10). The use of such systems is much more economical since four or nine images are produced

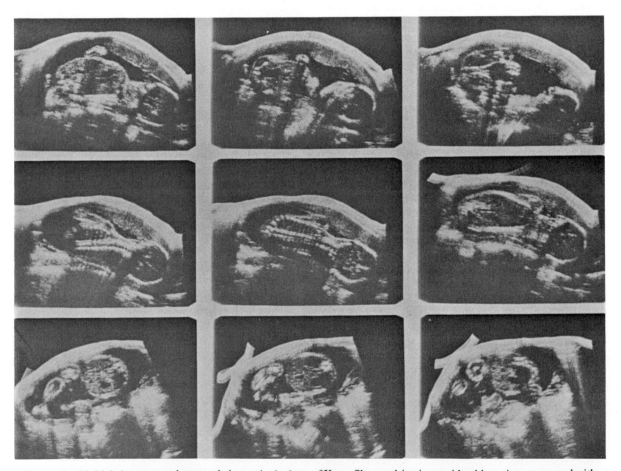

Fig. 1.10 Multiple images may be recorded on a single sheet of X-ray film resulting in considerable savings compared with the instant film.

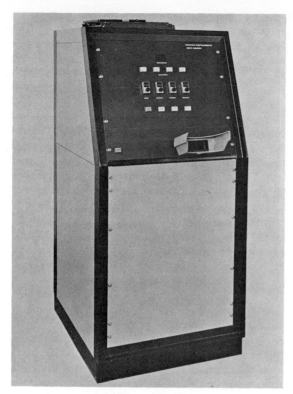

Fig. 1.11 Multiformat camera which may be used in conjunction with the scanners. Patient identification is a problem unless a character generator is used.

for less than $0.50 at current prices. Furthermore, storage with radiological files is facilitated, and this permits retrieval under the same system already in active use in the individual Radiology Department. Furthermore, X-ray film is tolerant to wide variations in contrast and intensity. Multiformat cameras may be rather large in dimension, although the floor space required can be minimized by standing the camera upright. Such a system is shown in Figure 1.11. Good photometry permits photography and precludes the necessity for multiple test plates. In one B-scanner commercially available, a multiformat camera is an optional integral part of the instrument.

Dynamic images

Modern ultrasound devices present the scans in video format and are usually viewed on a TV screen. It is obviously easy to store this information in video format on a tape recorder. For real-time systems this becomes essential and, with relatively little degradation in the resolution, the information may be recalled and static photography carried out on stopped frames. The least expensive systems are $\frac{1}{2}$ inch reel-to-reel video tape recorders, although the quality of the stopped frames is suboptimal due to tearing of the frames. By convention, professional television tape storage is carried out on a $\frac{3}{4}$ inch, and this will be adequate for most ultrasound studies, although some of the more sophisticated real-time phased array systems are deemed to require 1 inch tape to preserve adequately the quality of the image.

Video inversion

There is a sharp difference between the practice of most American radiologists and that of the European radiologists. In America most ultrasonologists have become accustomed to using a white background and the ultrasound image is recorded in black. Most Europeans, in contrast, have retained a black background and the image is then written in white. This is more compatible with the usual presentation of radiographs. From the author's experience, it appears that contour information can be adequately displayed by either format. However, when subtle differences of consistency must be recognized, it seems distinctly advantageous to use a background which does not flood the retina. This is demonstrated by Figures 1.12A and B, which show a subtle change in the consistency, in this case indicating metastatic disease. This is less easy to identify using a white background since the small difference in the brightness of the recorded echoes is frequently missed by the eye when faced with a bright background. At this medical center, it is routine for all ultrasound images to be recorded with black backgrounds, and we believe that this has led to much higher accuracy in detecting metastatic disease in the liver for the reasons that are apparent from the figures.

Real time ultrasound systems

Ultrasound B-mode scanning results in a two-dimensional display through soft tissue. If such images can be formed rapidly, and the position of an organ at any instant in time displayed virtually instantaneously, sequential presentation of these images on a nonstorage display system will permit the organ movement to be viewed in real-time. The limiting factors devolve from the rate of data acquisition, and this is directly imposed by immutable physical laws based on the velocity of sound in tissues. The basic time constants of short-pulse echo systems have already been considered; the exposure regime consists of microsecond pulses of ultrasound separated by intervals of 1000 μs giving a pulse repetition frequency (PRF) of 1000 per second. Since echoes from one pulse must not overlap those from a succeeding pulse, all echoes must have been received and died away within the 1000 μs interval between adjacent transmitted pulses. Since the velocity of sound in tissues is approximately 1500 MS^{-1}, the maximum travel of a sound wave in 1 ms is 150 cm, and this represents the distance for the round trip to and from the

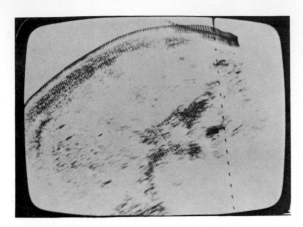

Fig. 1.12A Transverse B-mode ultrasonogram of the liver in a patient with metastatic disease using a white background format. It may be erroneously concluded that there is an echogenic metastasis situated posteriorly.

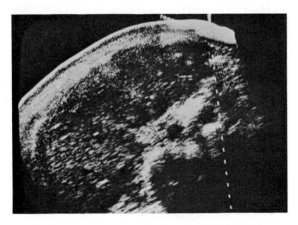

Fig. 1. 12B Shows the same section as that seen in Figure 1.12A with a black background format. The echogenic area posteriorly is now easily recognized as normal liver tissue, and the metastatic area is the more homogeneous tissue anterior to it.

reflector. It follows that the speed of sound in tissues limits the depth which may be displayed to 75 cm using a pulse-repetition frequency of 1000 per second. This depth is considerably more than is required in the clinical situation, or indeed allowed by tissue attenuation using current energy levels of the incident ultrasound beam. In the examination of most average-sized adults, 19 to 20 cm is the minimum distance required for depth penetration so that, if necessary, the pulse-repetition frequency of 1000 per second could be increased to 4000 pulses per second, which would reduce the tissue depth capable of being examined to approximately 19 cm.

For practical purposes, it is possible to obtain 4000 lines of data per second, and how these are divided can

be varied. For example, if an object is moving only slowly in time or if a rapid scan of an organ is required between cardiac pulsations, a high-resolution 1000 line scan can be completed in 0.25 seconds. If the object is rapidly moving and relatively flicker-free, real-time imaging is required; up to 50 frames per second must be utilized and each of these will only contain 80 data lines. With these limited data lines, the resolution that may be obtained is dependent upon the field of view. If the field of view is narrow, then 80 data lines may be entirely adequate to display the moving object, whereas if a large field of view is utilized, the individual data lines become separated and the apparent resolution degraded. This is demonstrated in Figures 1.13A and B, which show how a decrease in the field of view increases the data density and the apparent resolution.

From these considerations it is obvious that real-time scanning is achieved by the rapid sequential formation of individual B-scans. To produce a real-time scan, the ultrasound beam must be moved rapidly either in an arc or in a linear movement. For mechanical reasons, it is impractical to produce a linear movement of the transducer at high velocities so that the beam is moved by electronic rather than mechanical means. For a sector scan, the ultrasound beam may be moved either mechanically, by rocking the transducer, or electronically, by steering the ultrasound beam. These two methods of obtaining real-time scans are known as sector or linear scans. Sector scans may be produced by mechanical means or by electronic sector scans. Linear electronic scans are produced by linear arrays.

Linear arrays
A linear array is a line of transducers, up to 64 in a single array, which are individually rather small and produce a total array of less than 10 cm in length. The transducers are sequentially activated starting at one end and progressively exciting the transducers in turn, effectively sweeping the ultrasound beam from one end of the linear array to the other and producing a tomogram the length of which is the same length as the linear array. Sequential excitation of each of the transducers along the array results in one tomogram, and the process may be repeated up to 30 frames per second. The design of transducers and the sequelae of using very small transducers have already been considered (Fig. 1.5A). The use of a very small transducer compared with the wavelength results in a rapidly divergent beam with consequent degradation of the lateral resolution. To increase the size of the ultrasound beam relative to the wavelength, a battery of four transducers are activated at any one instant in time and this produces less beam divergence. However, the beam is nearly 1 cm wide, and this will be the lateral resolution of these linear array systems. The transducers are activated in blocks so that

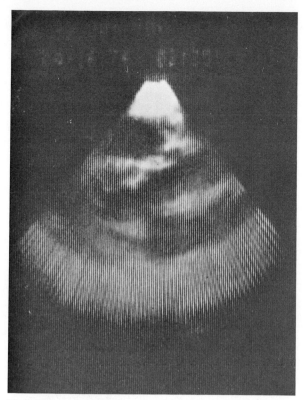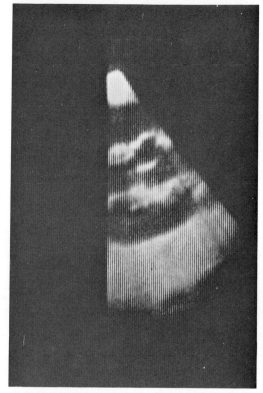

Fig. 1.13A Phased array sector scanner showing the effect of decreasing the angle of view. Figure 1.13A shows a large angle through the left outflow tract and there is separation of the individual data lines.

B A smaller angle of view approximates these data lines and enhances the resolution with which the left outflow tract and aortic valve are visualized.

transducers 1–4 are followed by 2–5, 3–6, 4–7, etc. This means that there will be 63 lines in each of the tomograms, and this is rather sparce data density for the long linear extent of the array.

Linear array systems do have the advantage that they are simple real-time systems which are relatively inexpensive, costing approximately $20,000 to $24,000 at current prices. For the reasons outlined above, the resolution is relatively poor so that these systems are predominantly suited for rapid screening purposes, especially in obstetrics where the placental position, fetal presentation, and size can be very simply and inexpensively determined. Due to the low-line density, spot films will be of extremely poor quality.

Sector scanning

Mechanical sector scanning. In a mechanical sector scanning system, the transducer is rapidly rocked through a small arc, producing a serial sector tomogram in one direction and then the other. The limitations of such a system devolve from the mechanics, since the transducer head needs to be moved rapidly in a smooth

manner without any lateral deviation. Such a system has been described by Griffith and Henry (1974), and clinical evaluation has shown the instrument to be valuable in assessing some types of congenital heart disease (Henry, Griffith, Michaelis *et al.*,1975).

Electronic sector scanner. Electronic sector scanners are more sophisticated instruments in which there is an array of transducers, and these transducers are activated at slightly different times such that the ultrasound beam is emitted at a definite angle from the transducer face (Fig. 1.14A). For the subsequent transmitted pulse, the excitation process is less delayed so that the ultrasound beam is more nearly perpendicular to the transducer face, while eventually there is no delay between activation of each transducer and the ultrasound beam is perpendicular to the transducer face (Fig. 1.14B). A further delay in the other direction enables the ultrasound beam to be swept laterally in the opposite direction (Fig. 1.14C). The entire delay in the excitation process results in the ultrasound beam being electronically swept through an arc or sector scan, and this is achieved rapidly without the limitations imposed by mechanical oscillation of the transducer head. These

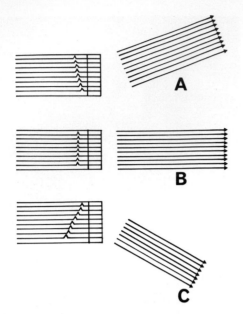

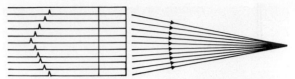

Fig. 1.15 In a phased array of transducers a suitable delay in the excitation process produces an ultrasound beam which is focused at a given distance from the transducer faces. The delay period can be infinitely varied to produce a focus at any given distance from the transducer face. This results in electronic focusing of a phased array system.

Fig. 1.14A A schema to show a phased array of transducers in which the excitation process is serially delayed. This results in an ultrasound wave leaving the transducer at an acute angle to it.

B An array of transducers which, excited at the same instant of time, gives rise to a wave front spreading out perpendicular to the transducer face.

C An array of transducers with the excitation process delayed in the opposite direction to produce a wave form spreading out at an angle to the transducer face. The sequential variation in the delay process sweeps the beam electronically from one side of the transducer to the other. This constitutes electronic sector scanning using a phased array system.

transducer systems are known as phased arrays. Systems using this principle tend to be highly expensive because of the technology involved in delaying the excitation process, these delay lines being extremely expensive.

Electronic focusing

Using the principle of the delay line, not only may an ultrasound beam be swept through a sector scan, but also the beam may be electronically focused at any desired depth, as shown in Figure 1.15. This principle is used in the most sophisticated real-time heart scanner currently available commercially. Unfortunately, the complexity of the system becomes sufficient to warrant a medium-sized computer to control the delay line system alone, so that the hardware is extremely expensive. Furthermore, it must be recalled that this type of electronic focusing is only achieved at present in one plane, so that the practical advantage of such systems over the less expensive fixed-focus systems achieved by simple acoustic lenses has yet to be evaluated. Much of the inordinate cost of real-time phased array systems is currently due to the cost of delay lines, and it seems

probable that in the near future these components will be replaced with inexpensive charge couple devices, which, together with the rapidly decreasing cost of computers, suggest that future technological advances will be towards highly sophisticated real-time phased array systems.

REFERENCES

Campbell, S. and Wilkin, D.: Ultrasonic measurement of fetal abdomen circumference in the estimation of fetal weight. *Br. J. Ob. Gynaec.*, **82**, 689–697, 1975.

Carlsen, E.N. and Filly, R.A.: Newer ultrasonographic anatomy in the upper abdomen: I. The portal and hepatic venous anatomy. *J. Clin. Ultrasound*, **4**, 85–90, 1976.

Donald, I., McVicar, J. and Brown, T.G.: Investigation of abdominal masses by pulsed ultrasound. *Lancet*, **1**, 1188–1194, 1958.

Fields, S. and Dunn, F.: Correlation of echographic vizualizability of tissue with biological composition and physiological state. Letter to the editor. *J. Acoust. Soc. Am.*, **54**, 809–812, 1973.

Filly, R.A. and Carlsen, E.N.: Newer ultrasonographic anatomy in the upper abdomen: II. The major systemic veins and arteries with a special note on localization of the pancreas. *J. Clin. Ultrasound*, **4**, 91–96, 1976.

Griffith, J.M. and Henry, W.L.: A sector scanner for real-time two-dimensional echocardiography. *Circulation*, **49**, 1147–1152, 1974.

Henry, W.L., Griffith, J.M., Michaelis, L.L. *et al.*: Measurement of mitral orifice area in patients with mitral valve disease by real-time, two-dimensional echocardiography. *Circulation*, **51**, 827–831, 1975.

Kossoff, G.: Display techniques in ultrasound pulse echo investigations: a review. *J. Clin. Ultrasound*, **2**, 61–72, 1974a.

Kossoff, G.: Ultrasonic visualization of the uterus, breast and eye by gray scale echography. *Proc. Royal Soc. Med.*, **67**, 135–140, 1974b.

Leopold, G.R.: Gray scale ultrasonic angiography of the upper abdomen. *Radiol.*, **117**, 665–617, 1975.

Taylor, K.J.W., Carpenter, D.A. and McCready, V.R.: Gray scale echography in the diagnosis of intrahepatic disease. *J. Clin. Ultrasound*, **1**, 284–287, 1973.

Taylor, K.J.W., Carpenter, D.A., McCready, V.R. *et al.*: Gray scale ultrasound imaging: the anatomy and pathology of the liver. *Radiol.*, **119**, 415–423, 1976.

Taylor, K.J.W. and McCready, V.R.: A clinical evaluation of gray scale ultrasonography. *Br. J. Radiol.*, **49**, 244–252, 1976.

2. Practical aspects of ultrasound scanning

The production of a technically adequate ultrasound tomogram is a prerequisite for proper interpretation and accurate diagnosis. All too frequently, a radiologic technician is co-opted as an ultrasound technician without further training, and this results in suboptimal scans, poor diagnostic accuracy, and ill repute for the modality. These difficulties are compounded when the interpreting physician is also a novice to the ultrasound technique and is therefore unable to suggest the means by which the technical quality can be improved.

The neophyte to ultrasound technology may find that a large percentage of his patients appear to have too much air in the gut to permit a diagnostically adequate scan. With more experience, most of these patients can be scanned by adoption of certain scanning techniques. In over 90% of patients, good scans can be obtained through the upper abdomen. In all patients, pelvic scans can be obtained using the bladder as an acoustic window which, when distended, displaces air-containing bowel from the pelvic cavity. The midabdomen is obscured in the majority of normal patients unless patient preparation has been effected. However, in patients with appreciable masses, air-containing gut is usually deflected to permit visualization of the mass. In addition, midabdominal pathology is rare compared with upper abdominal and pelvic pathology except when related to gut. Such pathology is well imaged by standard radiological opacification procedures.

At the present stage in the development of ultrasound technology, the acquisition of good B-scans is an art, and skilled, experienced technicians are in great demand. Scans must be immediately interpreted by the technician or physician to decide the placement of further sections for optimal display of any pathology. At the Yale–New Haven Hospital, technicians are trained for 12 months to achieve competence and experience in all applications of ultrasound scanning.

Although a stereotyped scanning process with multiple sections of every centimeter in the transverse and longitudinal planes is often advocated, such rigid adherence is wasteful of recording film and may result in large numbers of uninformative scans with scanty recordings of the pathological area. A well-trained technician should be capable of taking serial sections but also of recognizing and concentrating on any significant pathology. In areas of interest, sections should be taken in longitudinal, transverse, and oblique planes in every direction from which the pathology can be displayed.

In the following section, an attempt is made to aid the novice in scanning most effectively. In general, no patient preparation is carried out routinely, although patients are exhorted to use laxatives the night before examination if they are constipated. Preparation instructions for ultrasound examination are posted in each ward; these largely amount to fasting for a biliary tract examination and a full urinary bladder for pelvic examination. This list is shown in Table 2.1. Fasting is important before examination of the gallbladder since there may be difficulty in defining the gallbladder lumen unless it is dilated. Once the lumen is identified, multiple sections are taken through the gallbladder in search of gallstones. This search is greatly facilitated by the easy identification of the gallbladder. Furthermore, the inability of the gallbladder to distend in response to fasting may suggest a small shrunken organ which is incapable of physiological distention.

Table 2.1 Preparations required for ultrasound examinations

Gallbladder	Nothing by mouth, except water eight hours before examination
Heart	No special preparation
Kidney	No special preparation
Liver	No special preparation unless patient has been bedridden, when laxative may be required
Ob/Gyn	Patient must attend with a distended bladder
Pancreas	Patient should be scanned after light, bland meal, *not* carbonated liquid. Laxatives should be advised if there is any question of constipation
Spleen	No special preparation
Thyroid	No special preparation

Due to the high correlation between biliary tract disease and pancreatic disease, patients referred for pancreatic examination are optimally scanned when fasting to allow simultaneous assessment of the gallbladder. For liver examination, no preparation is essential, although it may be advantageous for the patient to have a light meal before scanning, since fasting patients tend to swallow more air than those who have eaten. Large meals may lead to confusing masses in the left upper quadrant which may require further scanning for elucidation. Alternately, if a mass is seen which could be abnormal or could be the distended stomach, distinction can be achieved if the patient drinks a carbonated beverage. If the mass is the stomach, the gas bubbles will cause immediate interference with the display of the mass.

Machine settings

As in radiological techniques, different parameters of dosage are required for different patients and for different examinations of the same patient. The major controls of importance in the acquisition of diagnostic ultrasound scans are the overall gain control and the TGC characteristics. The gain control must be set so that the normal internal structure of tissues is displayed, and the TGC must be adjusted so that the internal structure of normal tissue is evenly written. It must be recalled that the TGC is an electronic compensation for tissue attenuation. Thus, when optimally adjusted, the effects of normal tissue attenuation are no longer apparent. The principles given here are applicable to other organs, but the liver is chosen as an example.

The display of the internal structure of the liver demands the best instrumentation for its adequate demonstration. The liver is rather homogeneous on ultrasound examination, so that only low-level echoes emanate from within it. If these are properly processed, the normal internal structure will be evenly displayed. For speed, the appropriate gain and TGC characteristics can be adjusted while the operator monitors these adjustments on the A-scan. When a beam of ultrasound is transmitted through the liver by placing the ultrasound transducer under the right costal margin and directing the beam towards the head, a characteristic A-scan should be seen when the TGC and gain controls are optimally set. This is shown in Figure 2.1A. An initial transmit pulse is seen (I), and a large distal echo (D) indicates the position of the diaphragm. This distal echo can be observed to move with respiration. The substance of the liver returns echoes of lower amplitude, less than one-half of the amplitude of the diaphragmatic echo. Occasional higher level echoes are seen in the normal liver when the beam passes through the vicinity of the porta hepatis. However, most of the intrahepatic echoes are of similar low amplitude. Assuming that the liver is a homogeneous organ with similar interfaces throughout its substance, when all these reflectors produce echoes of equal amplitude, then the equipment is correctly compensating for tissue attenuation. a B-scan (see below) will result in a tomogram in which the intrahepatic echoes are equally distributed, as seen in Figure 2.1B.

If there is insufficient overall gain there will be very small echoes from within the liver, as seen on the A-scan.

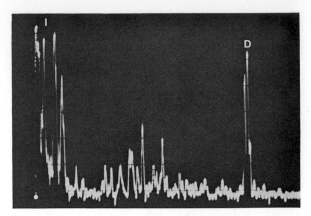

Fig. 2.1A A-scan through the normal liver with the TGC optimally adjusted. The initial transmit pulse (I) is of large amplitude and there is a large distal echo which indicates the position of the diaphragm (D). Between these extremes there are low-level echoes emanating from the intrahepatic structures with occasional high echoes in the region of the porta hepatis. All of the smaller echoes are of similar amplitude.

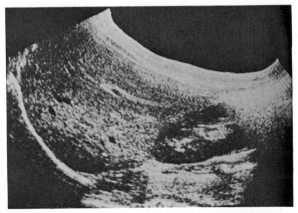

Fig. 2.1B A B-mode ultrasound scan through the right lobe of the liver shows the diaphragm above the liver and the right kidney on the posterior aspect of the liver. Note that the echoes are of similar amplitude throughout the liver parenchyma, although the deepest part of the liver adjacent to the diaphragm shows insufficient gain.

When a B-scan is performed, there will be insufficient display of the internal liver parenchyma (Fig. 2.2). This is the most common failure in liver scanning and detracts from the major advantage of the gray scale technique, which is the increased signal-to-noise ratio. On such inadequate scans, metastatic disease, small abscesses, and diffuse parenchymal abnormality are all likely to be missed. The display of the normal parenchyma is essential before defects of the fine anatomy can be appreciated or abnormal patterns can be recognized which indicate diffuse disease.

Conversely, excessive overall gain, as shown in Figure

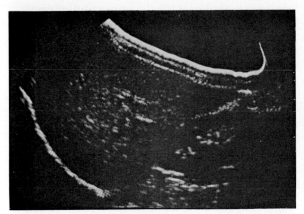

Fig. 2.2 B-mode scan through the right lobe of the liver and right kidney shows insufficient overall gain, so that there is inadequate display of the liver parenchyma, and only contour information of the size and shape of the liver and kidneys is apparent.

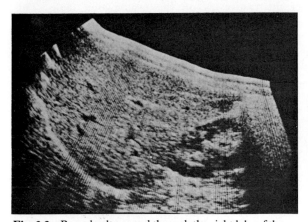

Fig. 2.3 B-mode ultrasound through the right lobe of the liver and kidney showing excessive gain. The parenchyma is displayed, but any abnormal areas, for example those due to homogeneous metastases, would be amplified sufficiently to simulate normal liver tissues.

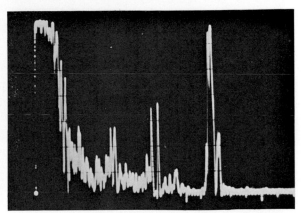

Fig. 2.4A A-mode scan through the liver showing the small intrahepatic echoes, which are larger anteriorly than posteriorly. This shows improper TGC adjustment with excessive gain anteriorly and insufficient gain posteriorly. The front gain should be reduced until the front echoes are of the same amplitude as the deeper echoes and the overall gain increased until the scan resembles that seen in Figure 2.1B.

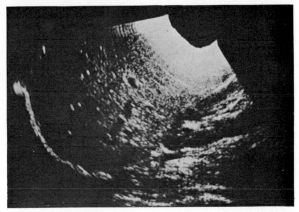

Fig. 2.4B B-mode scan with TGC adjusted as seen in Figure 2.4A. There is insufficient TGC to adequately demonstrate the deeper parts of the liver, indicating inadequate compensation for tissue attenuation.

2.3, overwrites the liver parenchyma. "Bleeding" may occur both from the viewing screen and during photography—causing spatially small, high intensity echoes to be increased in size and thereby seriously degrading the resolution. Of equal importance, metastatic disease of the liver will be missed since the difference in amplitude between tumor and normal liver may be only a few dB. With the compression-amplification systems used in gray scale, such differences in small echoes are exaggerated in the signal processing (see Fig. 1.7) but minimized when they are amplified by high gain.

Incorrect adjustment of the TGC will lead to nonuniform display of the hepatic parenchyma. There may be insufficient far gain due to tissue attenuation. The resulting A-scan is seen in Figure 2.4A. Note that the distal echoes are too small compared with the near echoes. The resulting B-scan shows a defect of the deep hepatic parenchyma which is purely due to poor technique and does not indicate a pathological space-occupying mass replacing the normal structure (Fig. 2.4B). Either the far gain can be increased, or the overall gain can be increased and the front gain decreased until the A-scan is similar to that shown in Figure 2.1A. Alternatively, there may be insufficient gain for the near echoes. The A-scan (Fig. 2.5A) shows that the anterior echoes are smaller than the deep ones, and this is reflected in the B-scan (Fig. 2.5B). Increasing the near gain may result in all the echoes being overamplified, so that the overall gain is decreased until the intrahepatic

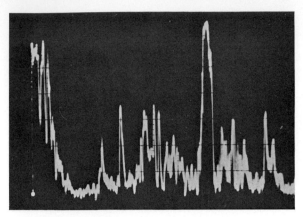

Fig. 2.5A A-mode scan through the liver showing inappropriate TGC with very small intrahepatic echoes anteriorly and larger echoes posteriorly. The front TGC should be increased and the overall gain decreased until the structure is written as in Figure 2.1B.

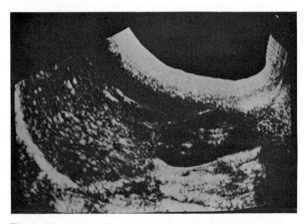

Fig. 2.5B A B-mode scan shows the right lobe of the liver and kidney with inappropriate TGC as seen in Figure 2.5A. The echoes from the superficial parts of the liver are inadequately amplified and the anterior TGC needs to be increased.

echoes are one-half to one-third the amplitude of the diaphragmatic echo. The final result in a normal liver must be the production of a scan showing normal structure which is evenly distributed throughout the liver. These comments relate to the normal liver and experience is rapidly gained in the characteristics of the normal liver. It will be noted in some patients that there are abnormally high-level echoes through the liver at low gain settings and that the usual TGC curve is totally insufficient. Mental note must be taken of any adjustments in gain that are required to compensate for correction of such abnormal liver, since this change in attenuation is indicative of a diffuse pathological process (p. 39).

Scanning techniques for the upper abdomen

Using a series of longitudinal and transverse scans with the patient in the supine position, an upper abdominal examination includes the liver, the gallbladder, the biliary tree, the great vessels, and the right kidney. Thus, the technique for scanning each of these organs is similar. First, a coupling medium must be used to ensure good transmission of the ultrasound beam into the patient. Although a number of proprietary gels are commercially available, these have only one advantage in that they are water soluble. They are therefore used preferentially in patients who are very sick and who will be unable to bathe immediately after the application of the oil. For all other patients, paraffin (mineral) oil is used. This is much less expensive than the gel media and is functionally superior. Whereas the gel tends to dry rapidly and impede ultrasonic transmission, paraffin oil remains liquid and thus ensures excellent contact. Paraffin oil does, however, dissolve the rubber coverings of the mattresses on the examination table. This problem can be overcome by covering the mattress with polythene.

When the area to be scanned has been liberally smeared with oil, the transducer is applied to the skin and the machine set according to the considerations in the preceding paragraph. The orientations of scans have now been standardized for both ultrasound and X-ray computerized tomographic body scanning. By convention a transverse section is viewed as though from the patient's feet. Thus, the patient's right side is displayed on the left of the TV screen as viewed by the operator facing the screen. This will involve the operator standing on the patient's right side with the patient facing away from the viewing screen. This has two advantages: the patient cannot see any obvious defect which appears on the screen and the transducer is available to the operator's right hand. The correct hold for the transducer is shown in Figure 2.6. The barrel of the transducer rests against the flexor surface of the finger pulps; the little finger tip lies next to the transducer face and locates intercostal spaces or the costal margin and so guides the transducer into the correct scanning position. The thumb is placed in apposition with the near side of the barrel of the transducer. With such a hold, the transducer is firmly under the control of the hand and movement is effected from the wrist. A common error is to hold the top of the transducer between the finger and the thumb like a pen (Fig. 2.7). There is insufficient control over the transducer when held in this position, so that the scan is not performed in a smooth fashion. In addition, the little finger is not available near the transducer tip to guide it into an optimal scanning location such as the intercostal space.

The transducer is placed immediately below the right

18

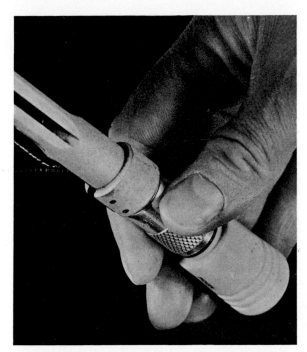

Fig. 2.6 When the transducer is correctly held, the barrell of the transducer rests against the flexor aspects of the fingers and the thumb rests on the other side of the transducer. The smallest finger is in contact with the skin and is used to continually monitor the amount of oil on the patient's skin and to guide the transducer into intercostal spaces or to place the transducer in the immediate subcostal position.

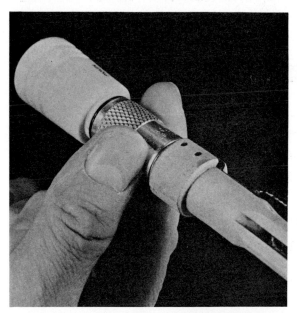

Fig. 2.7 Incorrect hold of the transducer between thumb and index finger. There is poor control of the movement of the transducer and the little finger is not available to monitor the state of the skin or to note the characteristics of any palpable mass.

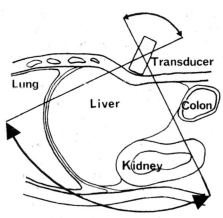

Fig. 2.8 Schema to show the position of the transducer for a subcostal scan in the paramedian plane. Access to the liver is limited by the costal margin above, the aerated lung above the diaphragm, and air in the colon below the liver. The combination of deep inspiration and contraction of the rectus abdominis muscle crowds the upper abdomen and displaces the air-containing colon, as well as bringing the liver as far as possible below the costal margin.

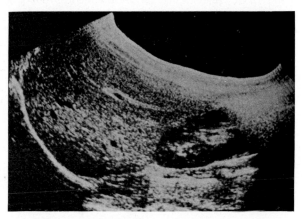

Fig. 2.9 Resulting B-mode scan of right lobe of the liver and kidney produced by single pass movement of the transducer, shown schematically in Figure 2.8.

costal margin with the transducer face pointing towards the patient's head. This is shown schematically in Figure 2.8. The transducer is then rotated in a smooth arc, adjusting the rate of travel to that required to write normal detailed intrahepatic anatomy (Fig. 2.9). The problems of upper abdominal scanning are well demonstrated in the schematic figure. The liver is limited above by air-containing lungs, anteriorly by the coastal margin, and inferiorly by air in the colon. The transducer must be placed immediately below the costal margin and the patient is instructed to inspire deeply. This brings the liver as inferior as possible and under the transducer face. At the same time, the patient is requested to contract the upper abdominal musculature which, together with the diaphragmatic contraction, crowds the upper abdomen and deflects the transverse colon downwards in most patents in whom the transverse colon has mobility on the mesocolon. This combination of inspiration and abdominal muscle contraction is critical in a number of patients and produces successful scanning in perhaps 10% of patients in whom the liver would otherwise be obscured. In other patients the transducer can be fitted into the intercostal spaces and small sector scans carried out, but the subcostal route produces optimal views of the liver.

The mechanical arm is then moved 1 cm to the right or left and the subcostal sector scan repeated. The resulting sections are demonstrated in the next chapter. These scans will cover the whole of the liver, the gallbladder lumen when the patient is fasting, the biliary tree, and at least the upper part of the right kidney. Permanent records are produced by photography of the slave monitor with Polaroid or other hard copy.

The mechanical arm is then moved into the transverse plane. In this plane it may be worthwhile to produce a compounded scan to obtain an overall impression of the organ size and contour on an axial tomogram. However, for the reasons stated in the preceding chapter (pp. 8–9), fine resolution is obtained only by single pass scans, whether they are sector or linear.

During transverse scanning, the subxiphoid sector scan and the intercostal scan are of particular value. The subxiphoid scan is shown schematically in Figure 2.10. The patient is requested to inspire deeply to bring the liver edge as inferior as possible to provide an acoustic window to the prevertebral region. The level of the transducer is immediately below the xiphoid process. The transducer is angulated acutely to the right and then rotated until it is perpendicular with the skin, moved across the epigastrium, and angled under the left subcostal margin. The resulting scan (Fig. 2.11) shows the great vessels, liver, kidneys and, in lower sections, the pancreas. Sections can be taken at an increasing distance below the xiphisternum but may frequently be limited by air in the gut. In such patients, these transverse scans may be supplemented by intercostal sector scans. This technique is shown schematically in Figure 2.12. The transducer is positioned in the right intercostal space. Small sector movements of the transducer result in excellent display of the right kidney, renal vessels, and the gallbladder, lying anterior to the right kidney (Fig. 2.13). The same technique may be used to display the left kidney (Fig. 2.12).

In conclusion, an attempt has been made in the initial chapters of this book to explain the principles involved in diagnostic ultrasound and, in particular, the gray scale modifications. The ability to display the non-specular, backscattered echoes from pulsating organs in the upper abdomen implies that compound scanning, which was essential on the older instrumentation, not only can be abandoned but *must* be abandoned if the optimum resolution is to be obtained. Precise planes of

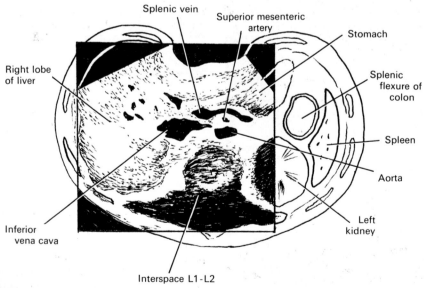

Fig. 2.10 Schema to show the movement of the transducer for a subxiphoid scan. The transducer is first rotated as far as possible to the right and then brought into the perpendicular position, moved across the epigastrium, and rotated to the left, producing as nearly as possible an axial tomogram. Note, however, that this is a single pass technique; thus the beam is incident on any point reflector on only one occasion and each point is registered in one position despite any subsequent movement.

scanning should be intelligently sought without strict adherence to a rigid routine. The use of such technique demands excellent anatomical knowledge of both physi- cian and technician, but assures superb resolution and the acquisition of unique information by a totally noninvasive method.

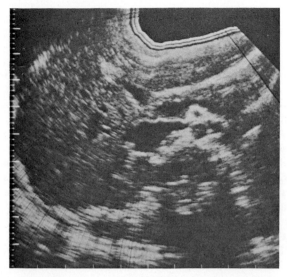

Fig. 2.11 Transverse axial tomogram produced by the single pass technique shown schematically in Figure 2.10. Note the fine resolution obtained by this technique despite biological motion.

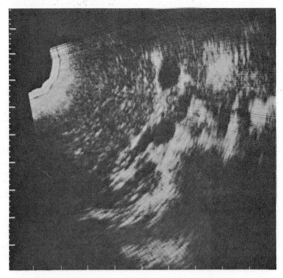

Fig. 2.13 This transverse sector scan through the intercostal space shows the right kidney and gallbladder displayed by the technique shown in Figure 2.12.

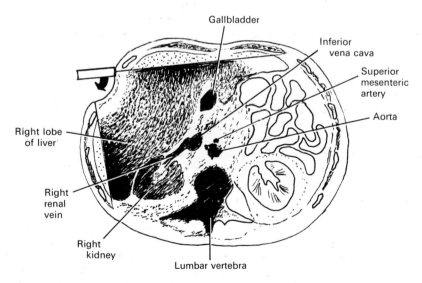

Fig. 2.12 Schema to show intercostal scans which present transverse tomograms through the right kidney, liver, and gallbladder. The renal vessels can be well displayed. The same technique may be used to produce a transverse tomogram through the left kidney.

3. Indications for scanning the liver and the upper abdomen

There is a very large number of clinical conditions in which ultrasonic examination of the upper abdomen may yield useful clinical information which, when supplemented by results of physical examination, may be diagnostic. These clinical conditions are too numerous to list, but nine general categories are considered and are summarized in Table 3.1. It is hoped that this will serve as a guide, for both referring physicians and potential ultrasonologists, to the type of patient in whom ultrasonic examination is likely to produce useful data.

Table 3.1 General categories of disease entities in which ultrasonic examination of the upper abdomen should be undertaken

1. Right upper quadrant mass
2. Constitutional symptoms, including loss of weight, malaise, fever of unknown origin
3. Right upper quadrant pain
4. Cholestatic jaundice
5. Metastatic workup
6. Equivocal or positive nuclear scan
7. Effect of hepatotoxic agents
8. Persistent pleural opacities of the right base
9. Congenital diseases affecting liver, kidney, pancreas, or spleen

Palpable upper abdominal masses

In any patient presenting with a palpable abdominal mass, ultrasound examination complements and supplements the findings of physical examination. The ultrasonologist has the unique advantage of being able to rapidly augment his clinical examination with tomographic sections of the palpated mass, and this significantly increases his experience and sensitivity by which abdominal masses are detected. Patients may be referred who appear clinically to have a right upper quadrant mass, while immediate ultrasound examination of the palpated tumor shows the lower part of the right kidney, which is frequently easily felt in thin patients, or a Riedel's lobe, so that these anatomical variations are easily differentiated from significant tumors. The ability to differentiate between solid and cystic masses by ultrasonic examination is also a valuable addition to the clinical examination since this frequently permits differentiation between benign and malignant propensity. Ultrasound also permits the relation of the mass to the surrounding organs to be satisfactorily delineated so that cystic masses within the liver may be differentiated from a hydrops of the gallbladder, renal cyst or hydronephrosis, pancreatic pseudocyst, or abscess cavity. Ultrasonic examination of solid masses always helps by determining the relation of the mass to the surrounding organs to indicate the organ of origin of the mass and, by its cross-sectional appearances, to suggest the pathological type of tumor, in particular whether it is neoplastic or inflammatory.

Constitutional disturbances

These may be indications for liver examination. In patients presenting with constitutional disturbances, including such nonspecific findings as malaise, weight loss, or fever of unknown origin, ultrasound may assist in excluding the responsible pathology such as liver abscess or liver metastasis, or may be diagnostic in imaging such pathology. Ultrasound is the modality of choice for the diagnosis of liver abscess, for which it is extremely accurate. However, abscesses may occasionally be misdiagnosed as simple cysts or necrotic tumors. In the diagnosis of the right subphrenic abscess, ultrasound is, in our experience, the most accurate modality, approaching 100 %. A left subphrenic abscess may be missed owing to the proximity to and confusion with fluid-containing gut, stomach, and spleen. An accuracy of only 90 % is achieved in the diagnosis of left subphrenic abscesses.

Right upper quadrant pain

Ultrasound is a potentially useful modality to investigate possible causes of right upper quadrant pain in a patient presenting without clinical signs. Pain associated with hydrops of the gallbladder or gallstones producing biliary sepsis are well imaged by ultrasonic examination of the right upper quadrant. An acute hydronephrosis producing right upper quadrant pain is also easily distinguished at the same examination. In addition, liver abscess, pancreatitis, and abdominal aneurysms are apparent.

Signs of liver failure, for example jaundice

Ultrasonic examination of the liver is always indicated in patients presenting with jaundice of the cholestatic type. The major problem in these patients is to differentiate between intrahepatic causes of cholestasis and extrahepatic biliary obstruction, which is characterized by dilatation of the whole biliary tree. Gray scale ultrasound is the most effective method for differentiating between these two diagnostic possibilities since it enables the physiological state of the biliary tree to be well displayed. Whereas the condition of the biliary tree as apparent on percutaneous cholangiography depends upon the amount and pressure with which the contrast medium was injected, the physiological condition of the biliary vessel as demonstrated by ultrasound allows much subtler degrees of biliary distention to be recognized. In many of these patients the precise anatomical site of the obstruction is seen, as for example in biliary obstruction due to a carcinoma of the head of the pancreas. In those patients with intrahepatic cholestasis, the recognition of diffuse pathology such as cirrhosis or metastatic disease frequently enables the cause of hepatic failure to be defined.

Metastatic workup
In patients presenting with primary tumors, many surgeons routinely request a technetium polyphosphate bone scan and an isotopic liver scan before proceeding to radical surgery. In the experience of the author, ultrasonic examination of the liver has proved to be a more sensitive modality to detect early metastatic disease (Smith, Taylor, McCready *et al.*, 1976). Ultrasound has also been successfully used for the early detection of lymphoma in both the liver and the spleen in the preoperative staging of Hodgkin's disease and non-Hodgkin's lymphoma. In this application ultrasound proved superior to isotope techniques (Glees, Taylor, Gazet *et al.*, 1977).

Differentiation of positive or equivocal nuclear scans
Since in the large majority of patients ultrasound permits differentiation of nonspecific cold areas on isotope scans into those due to cysts, abscesses, or metastases, the method can be used to increase the specificity of the liver investigation. In addition, in a relatively large number of patients with equivocal nuclear scans which may be due to anatomical variation or significant pathology, ultrasound also permits differentiation (Taylor, Sullivan, Rosenfield *et al.*, 1977).

Effect of hepatotoxic agents
In the examination of the upper abdomen, ultrasound permits examination of the effects of hepatotoxic agents, the most common example of which is alcohol. Fatty infiltration in cirrhosis presents characteristic ultrasound findings. The development of portal hypertension may be implied by observations of the portal vein, which becomes enlarged and tortuous, and congestive splenomegaly can be quantitated and monitored. The method has also been evaluated in a preliminary study to monitor the changes after exposure to monovinyl chloride (Taylor, Williams, Smith *et al.*, 1975).

Persistent pleural opacities at the right base
Ultrasound examinations of the upper abdomen should be carried out for persistent pleural opacities of the right lung field base. Sections through the liver in the parasagittal plane reveals the right hemidiaphragm, and scans of inspiration and expiration confirm diaphragmatic movement even when this is not apparent on fluoroscopy due to lung field opacities. Furthermore, the method allows differentiation between consolidation of the lung and surrounding pleural effusion and also localizes the fluid for aspiration. Occasionally a pleural effusion may be due to a right subphrenic abscess, and a right subphrenic abscess is very accurately diagnosed by the ultrasound technique.

Congenital diseases
Patients with family histories of abnormality in the organs of the right upper quadrant can be easily scanned and screened using the ultrasound technique. In the state of Connecticut, there are some 30 families who are involved with polycystic disease, and ultrasonic examination of all relatives of affected members detects the cystic changes not only in the kidneys but also throughout the liver. Similarly, patients predisposed by metabolic disease to the formation of gallstones can be easily investigated, and the siblings of patients with congenital hepatic fibrosis can be detected before there is risk of progression of the disease to portal hypertension and esophageal varices.

In the following pages, examples of many of these entities will be described and the differential diagnoses considered.

REFERENCES

Glees, J.P., Taylor, K.J.W., Gazet, J.C. *et al.*: Accuracy of grey-scale ultrasonography of the liver and spleen in Hodgkin's Disease and other lymphomas compared with isotope scans. *Clin. Radiol.*, **28**, 233–238, 1977.

Smith, I.E., Taylor, K.J.W., McCready, V.R. *et al.*: *Clin. Oncology*, **2**, 47–53, 1976.

Taylor, K.J.W., Sullivan, D., Rosenfield, A.T. *et al.*: Grey-scale ultrasound and isotope scanning: complementary techniques for imaging the liver. *Am. J. Roentgenol.*, **128**, 277–281, 1977.

Taylor, K.J.W., Williams, D.M.J., Smith, P.M. *et al.*: Grey-scale ultrasonography for monitoring industrial exposure to hepatotoxic agents. *Lancet*, **1**, 1222, 1975.

4. The liver

4.1 Normal anatomy, longitudinal

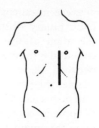

This parasagittal section 2 cm to the left of the midline shows the aorta posteriorly and the normal liver substance anteriorly. In the upper figure two branches can be seen originating from the anterior aspect of the aorta and passing inferiorly. These are the celiac and superior mesenteric arteries. The inferior continuation of the celiac axis seen running parallel to the superior mesenteric artery is probably the gastroduodenal artery.

In the lower figure, the aorta is again seen posteriorly, and anterior to the aorta is the superior mesenteric vein. The bulbus termination of the superior mesenteric vein is due to its fusion with the splenic vein to form the portal vein. The left lobe of the liver is seen, limited by the chest wall anteriorly and the central tendon of the diaphragm above.

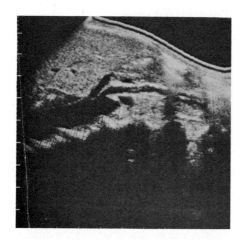
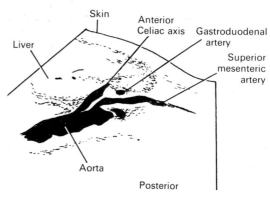

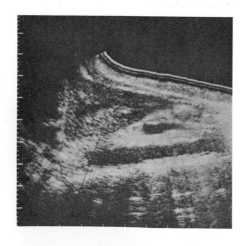
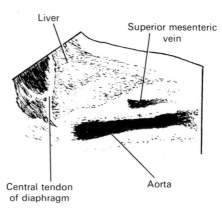

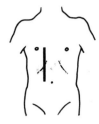

4.2 Normal anatomy, longitudinal

The upper figure is a parasagittal section 2 cm to the right of the midline showing the inferior vena cava posteriorly. The lumen of the inferior vena cava varies markedly with respiratory and cardiac cycles. Again, the normal liver consistency is seen anterior to the vena cava, and the liver is limited anteriorly by the abdominal wall and superiorly by the central tendon of the diaphragm.

The lower figure shows a similar section but cuts the portal vein as it runs along the free edge of the lesser omentum from its formation posterior to the neck of the pancreas to the porta hepatis. Note that the normal portal vein is relatively straight except for a sudden concavity at its termination. The right branch of the portal vein is well seen on transverse sections (see Fig. 4.4), and the portal vein radicles are characterized by highly reflective walls. The middle hepatic vein is seen draining into the inferior vena cava just below the diaphragm.

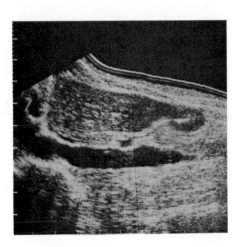

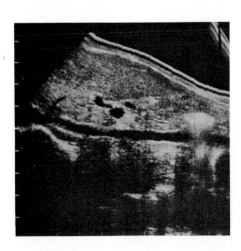

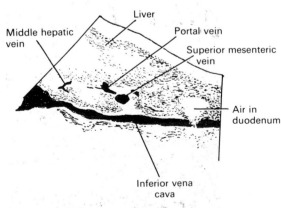

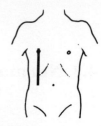

4.3 Normal anatomy, longitudinal

The upper figure shows a longitudinal scan 4 cm to the right of the midline, demonstrating the consistency of the liver. In this position, the liver is limited above by the right hemidiaphragm, anteriorly by the abdominal wall, and posteriorly by the right kidney—from which it is separated by the perirenal fat and fascia. These appear as a single highly reflective interface. This well-marked hepatorenal differentiation may be less obvious in very emaciated patients, as seen in Figure 4.6.

The lower figure shows a similar sagittal section taken after fasting, with the gallbladder lumen well displayed. The right branch of the portal vein is seen on transverse section and has highly reflective walls. The branches of the hepatic veins have thinner walls, and the bifurcations of the branches point towards the diaphragm.

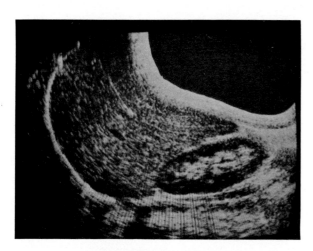

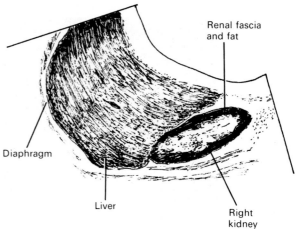

Renal fascia and fat

Diaphragm

Liver

Right kidney

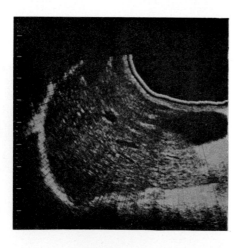

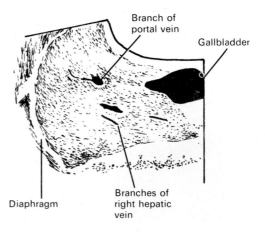

Branch of portal vein

Gallbladder

Diaphragm

Branches of right hepatic vein

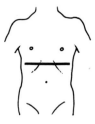

4.4 Normal anatomy, transverse

This transverse section through the upper abdomen (upper figure) shows the aorta and inferior vena cava with the celiac trunk originating from the aorta. The celiac trunk divides after about 2 cm into the splenic artery, passing towards the left, and the hepatic artery, which passes towards the right. The left gastric artery, which is the third branch of the celiac trunk, is not seen.

Anterior to the inferior vena cava, the portal vein is seen with the right branch of the portal vein extending out towards the right and dividing into anterior and posterior branches.

The lower figure shows a more limited sector scan at the same level, showing the celiac axis and its branches. Again, the right branch of the portal vein is seen.

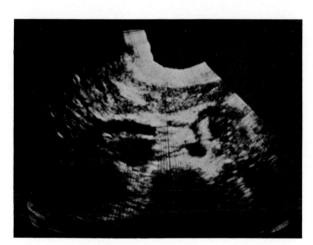

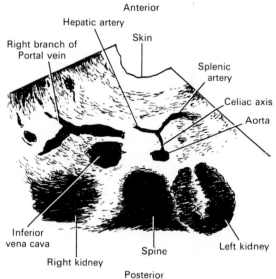

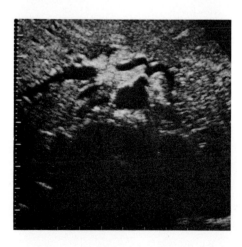

4.5 Normal anatomy, transverse

The upper figure shows a transverse sector scan with the transducer placed immediately below the xiphisternum. The liver consistency is well displayed and the right kidney is seen posteriorly. The aorta, inferior vena cava, and right branch of the portal vein are seen.

The lower ultrasonogram demonstrates a lower section 3 cm below the xiphisternum, again produced by a simple sector scan. As above, the right kidney is seen posterior to the liver, while the lumen of the gallbladder is seen anteriorly. The aorta and inferior vena cava are seen in the prevertebral position. The splenic vein passes around the prevertebral vessels, joining the superior mesenteric vein to form the portal vein, which is seen anterior to the inferior vena cava. The body and tail of the pancreas are anterior to the splenic vein. When distended, the stomach may be visualized in the upper quadrant and must be differentiated from significant space-occupying masses. A drink of water or a carbonated beverage may be used, as seen in Figure 12.7.

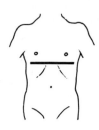

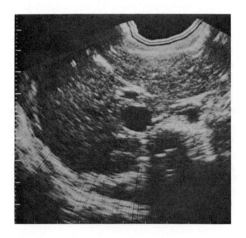

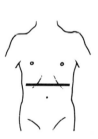

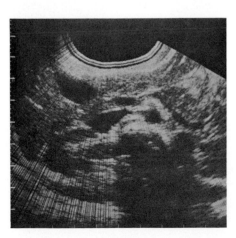

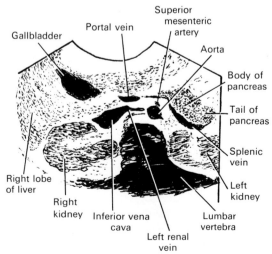

Gallbladder

Portal vein

Superior mesenteric artery

Aorta

Body of pancreas

Tail of pancreas

Splenic vein

Left kidney

Right lobe of liver

Right kidney

Inferior vena cava

Left renal vein

Lumbar vertebra

4.6 Normal anatomy—hepatorenal differentiation in thin patients

The right kidney is usually well differentiated from the liver (see Fig. 4.3). Usually the renal fascia is not separately imaged from the perirenal fat, so that the usual interface between the liver and kidney must be due to both the perirenal fascia and fat. This elderly male patient was a chronic alcoholic and was emaciated, with minimal body fat. The hepatorenal angle presents an unusual appearance.

The paramedian scan from the anterior aspect (upper figure) shows the right lobe of the liver and right kidney. The pyramids are well seen, so that the renal cortex and medulla are separately differentiated. The hepatorenal interface is barely defined.

Visualization of the liver and kidney from the posterior aspect (lower figure) confirms an unusually thin white interface between liver and kidney. These findings suggest that the normal perirenal fat contributes to the usual well-marked interface between the liver and kidney.

The presence of fat has a pronounced scattering effect on the ultrasound beam, and the lack of fat in this patient may account for the unusually good display of the renal pyramids.

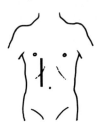

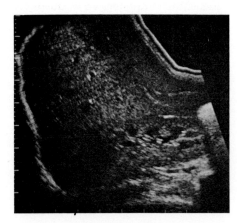

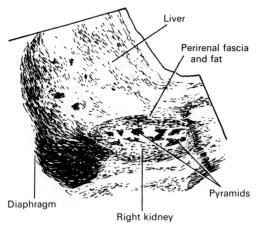

Liver

Perirenal fascia
and fat

Pyramids

Diaphragm

Right kidney

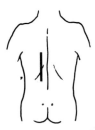

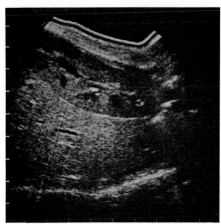

4.7 Congenital pathology—benign cyst

A. This isolated cyst was an incidental finding in a healthy volunteer. The fluid contents of the lesion are indicated by the excessive amplification of the structures distal to the lesion. The A-scan showed no evidence of echoes throughout the lesion.

B. A 48-year-old female presented with carcinoma of the breast, apparently stage 1. Routine preoperative isotope scanning showed a definite defect on the posterior view of the liver, indicating a space-occupying lesion, which was considered to be due to a metastasis. A paramedian ultrasonogram 6 cm to the right of the midline shows that there is a simple cystic mass, divided by a septum, lying above the right kidney. The flat A-scan confirms that there is no cellular debris and the walls are regular, and these appearances indicate a benign cyst. Metastases from breast in liver are frequently necrotic and cystic, but this is usually seen only after energetic treatment, and some solid metastases are always seen.

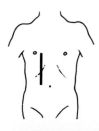

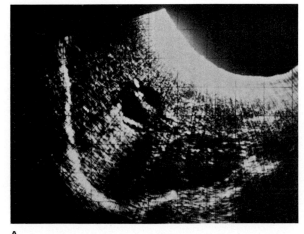

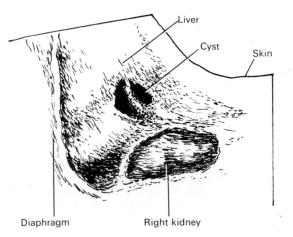

A

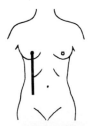

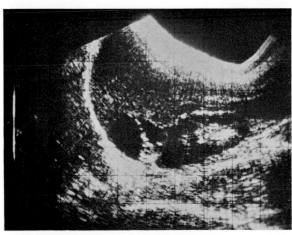

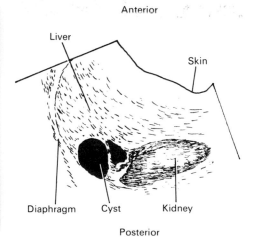

B

33

4.8 Congenital pathology—congenital polycystic disease

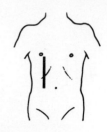

This 60-year-old patient was known to have a congenital polycystic disease, and other members of the patient's family were affected. A paramedian section through the right lobe of the liver shows gross cystic changes throughout the liver and right kidney so that these organs cannot be separately delineated.

Ultrasound has been successfully used at the Yale-New Haven Hospital to identify presymptomatic polycystic disease in the progeny of patients with established disease. Evidence to date suggests that ultrasound is a more sensitive modality for detecting polycystic disease than either conventional radiological techniques or computerized tomography.

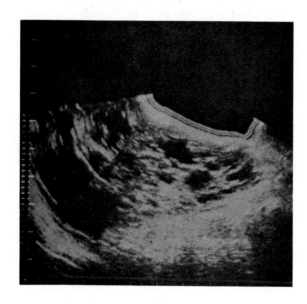

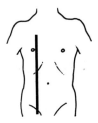

4.9 Congenital pathology—cavernous hemangiomata

This 24-year-old patient was referred for diagnosis with a palpable liver discovered on routine clinical examination. Isotope scanning revealed multiple space-occupying lesions, and the ultrasonogram is consistent with this. The paramedian section, taken 6 cm to the right of the midline, shows multiple small, highly homogeneous lesions throughout the liver substance. Many tumors simulate such homogeneous appearances. Biopsy was carried out at laparotomy and these lesions were found to be cavernous hemangiomata.

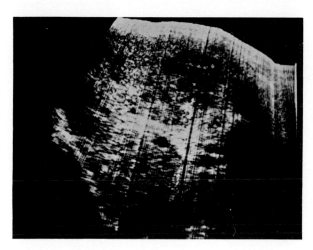
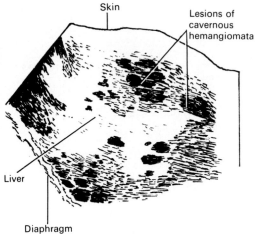

4.10 Congenital pathology—Hunter's syndrome

This 4-year-old child had gargoyle-like features and was referred for ultrasound examination to estimate the size of the abdominal organs. The transverse ultrasonogram of the liver (upper figure) shows a highly abnormal consistency with fine, high-level echoes, similar to that seen in fatty infiltration. In addition, there are linear reflective streaks. The longitudinal ultrasonogram (lower figure) shows the right lobe of the liver, which is enlarged to the right kidney. The abnormal consistency is again noted. These appearances are consistent with diffuse infiltration with mucopolysaccharide.

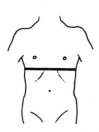

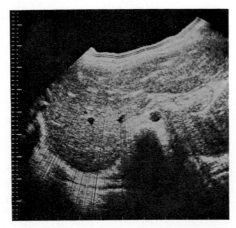

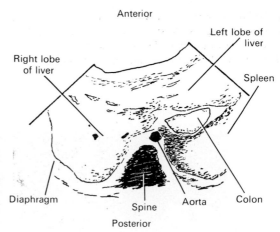

Anterior

Left lobe of
liver

Right lobe
of liver

Spleen

Diaphragm

Spine

Aorta

Colon

Posterior

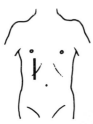

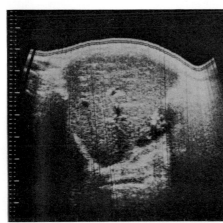

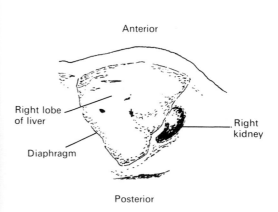

Anterior

Right lobe
of liver

Right
kidney

Diaphragm

Posterior

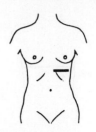

4.11 Congenital pathology—situs inversus viscerum

This 4-year-old girl with dextrocardia was referred for investigation of possible situs inversus viscerum. The transverse ultrasonogram of this very active child shows the liver filling the entire left side of the abdomen. The left hepatic vein and its branches are well seen draining into the inferior vena cava. Ultrasound is a rapid and highly accurate means for determining the position of soft abdominal and pelvic organs.

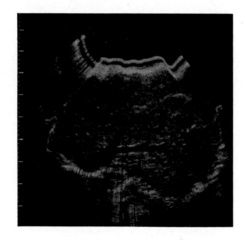

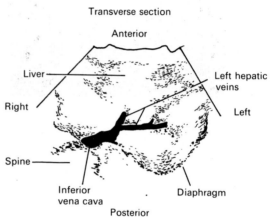

Transverse section

Anterior

Liver

Right

Spine

Inferior
vena cava

Posterior

Left hepatic
veins

Left

Diaphragm

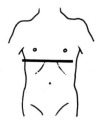

4.12 Congenital pathology—congenital hepatic fibrosis

This 16-year-old boy presented with hematemesis, and investigation revealed esophageal varices due to portal hypertension. He was admitted for portacaval anastomosis but postoperatively developed marked ascites, and right upper quadrant pain suggested the possibility of an abscess. He was referred for ultrasound investigation.

The transverse ultrasonogram performed at 1.6 MHz showed a liver identical to that seen in advanced cirrhosis (Fig. 4.41). Adjusting the TGC to reduce the

near gain and increasing the far gain (p. 17) resulted in this scan. Marked ascites is seen separating the liver from the abdominal wall, and the liver shows high-level echoes. The greatly increased attenuation has been overcome by the use of 1.6 MHz and by adjustment of the TGC.

The appearances are those of diffuse and severe intrahepatic fibrosis, and it is impossible to tell whether this is congenital in origin or acquired. No abscess cavity was visualized.

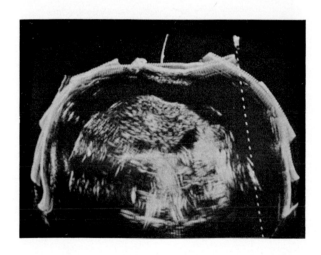

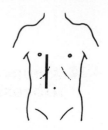

4.13 Congenital pathology—congenital hepatic fibrosis and Caroli's syndrome

This 3-year-old boy was referred for examination for attacks of fever and transient jaundice. The B-mode ultrasound examination shows a grossly abnormal liver consistency with abnormally high level intrahepatic echoes, well seen on the A-scan. (Compare this with the normal liver A-scan, p. 16.) Such findings are consistent with diffuse intrahepatic fibrosis which, in this child, is probably of congenital origin. Closer examination of the B-scan also shows multiple defects which represent cystic cavities and are consistent with Caroli's syndrome. This was confirmed by transhepatic cholangiography.

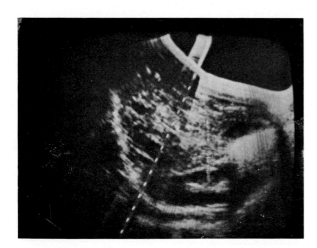

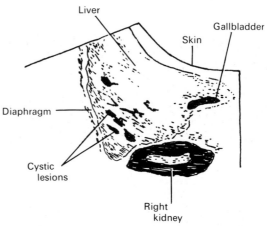

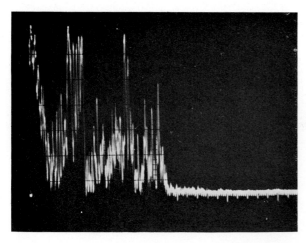

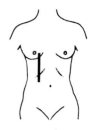

4.14 Inflammatory state—ascending cholangitis and subdiaphragmatic abscess

This 39-year-old female developed right upper quadrant pain and fever on her arrival in London from Jamaica. Immediate laparotomy revealed an empyema of the gallbladder, and at surgery the liver was noted to be friable. Postoperatively, the patient remained gravely ill and her fever persisted. She was referred for ultrasound examination to exclude or localize a hepatic abscess.

A paramedian ultrasonogram 6 cm to the right of the midline shows diffuse abnormality of the hepatic parenchyma with coarse, high-level flecks consistent with diffuse inflammatory changes. Immediately beneath the right hemidiaphragm is a homogeneous area replacing the liver parenchyma. Such a space-occupying mass in a liver showing inflammatory changes is indicative of an abscess. These appearances were therefore interpreted as ascending cholangitis with subdiaphragmatic abscess formation. The abscess was drained.

Ultrasound is a most effective means for diagnosing intrahepatic, right subphrenic, and right subhepatic abscesses. In these anatomical sites, ultrasonic investigation has proved 100% correct over the past three years of the author's experience. Left subphrenic abscesses may be missed owing to the juxtaposition of the stomach, colon, and spleen.

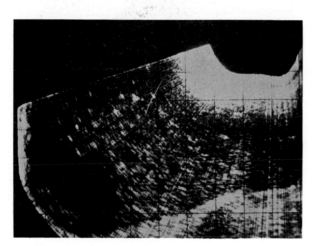

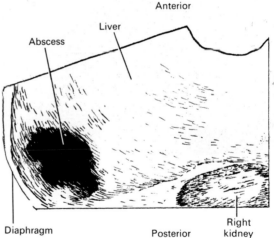

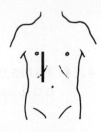

4.15 Inflammatory state—*E. coli* intrahepatic abscess

A 25-year-old male presented with a history of pyrexia of unknown origin and was referred for ultrasound examination to exclude a subphrenic or hepatic abscess. A paramedian ultrasonogram 6 cm to the right of the midline shows a large semifluid mass within the liver. Note that there are high-level echoes posterior to the lesion, indicating a low attenuation, while low-level echoes arise within the mass. A liver abscess was drained at surgery.

These appearances may be confused with those of a homogeneous tumor. The presence of a thick capsule surrounding a liquid collection is highly characteristic of a chronic liver abscess. Correct differentiation between metastasis and abscess has been achieved in 88 % of the author's series, despite similarity of appearances.

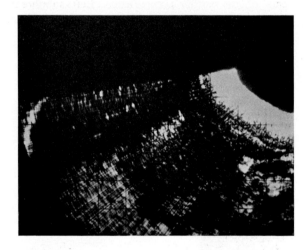

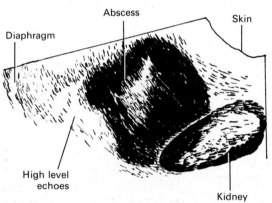

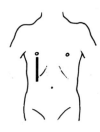

4.16 Inflammatory state—subhepatic abscess

This 18-year-old male was referred with fever of unknown origin and leucocytosis. Ultrasound examination was requested to exclude or localize an abdominal or pelvic abscess. Longitudinal sections through the liver and right kidney show an abnormal mass immediately below the liver, and this mass extends into the peritoneal space between the liver and right kidney (hepatorenal or Morison's pouch). The abnormal mass contains many internal echoes, indicating much cellular debris. The appearances are consistent with semifluid pus in this subhepatic abscess.

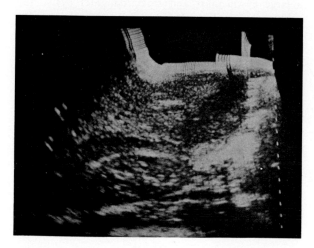

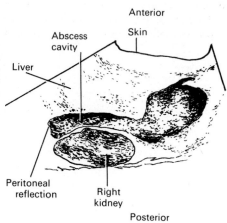

4.17 Inflammatory state—hydatid disease

A. A 60-year-old patient presented as a case of an unresolved pneumonia with a persistent opacity at the right base. The possibility of an underlying subphrenic abscess was raised and she was referred for ultrasonography. A paramedian scan is shown 8 cm to the right of the midline and large cystic masses are obvious. The diaphragm is not easily identified, and the liver substance is abnormal—showing irregular high-level echoes which suggest an inflammatory process. Both the consistency of the liver and the extension of disease above the diaphragm imply that this must be an inflammatory process and is consistent with hydatid disease. At surgery, multiple abscesses were found which had eroded through the diaphragm into the pleural space.

B. An Egyptian woman of 55 years presented with general malaise, and clinical examination revealed an enlarged liver. She was referred for ultrasound examination. The paramedian section taken 4 cm to the right of the midline shows an abnormal liver consistency with a large cystic mass and small daughter cysts. The gallbladder is well displayed, as is the right kidney. The appearance is that of hydatid disease of the liver.

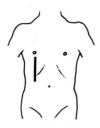

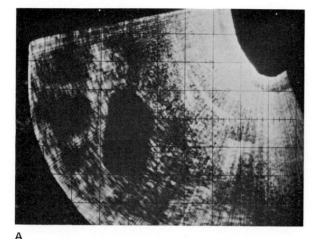

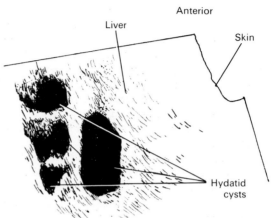

Anterior

Liver

Skin

Hydatid
cysts

A

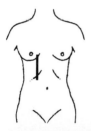

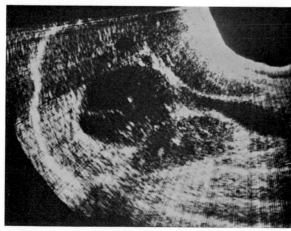

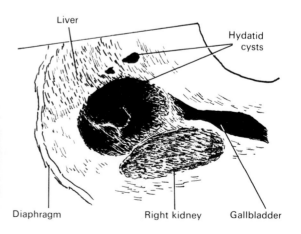

Liver

Hydatid
cysts

Diaphragm

Right kidney

Gallbladder

B

4.18 Tumor—homogeneous liver metastases

A 60-year-old woman presented with advanced metastatic disease and exploratory laparotomy revealed a retroperitoneal leiomyosarcoma with metastases to the liver. She was referred for ultrasound evaluation of the liver as a baseline prior to instituting chemotherapy.

The parasagittal ultrasonogram (upper figure) and transverse ultrasonogram (lower figure) reveal obvious defects of the normal liver consistency. These appearances are characteristic of untreated metastatic disease of the liver.

Both sarcomas and lymphomas tend to produce highly homogeneous (low echo-producing) metastases in the liver. Most carcinomas also produce homogeneous areas in the untreated patient, but the differences between metastatic areas and normal tissue may be small. Apart from this difference in echo amplitude, the metastases tend to produce a finer tissue consistency than the normal liver substance. Mucin-secreting adenocarcinomas of the colon and liver metastases in patients undergoing chemotherapy often show echogenic areas. In the author's experience, the overall accuracy of ultrasound examination of liver metastases is 92 %. However, detection of liver metastases by ultrasound does require the best instrumentation and considerable experience by the operator. Compared with isotope examination of the liver, ultrasound allows differentiation between significant pathology and anatomical variation (see Figs. 4.41–4.46).

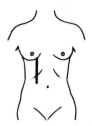

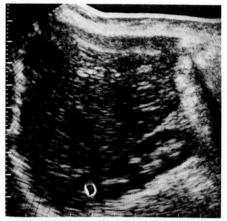

upper

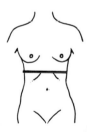

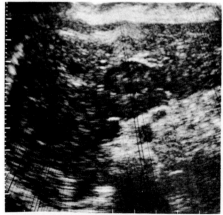

lower

4.19 Malignancy—echogenic liver metastases from carcinoma of the colon

An elderly man was referred for ultrasonic evaluation by his primary care physician because of malaise and hepatomegaly.

A. The longitudinal scan of the liver shows multiple areas of high-level echoes with irregular edges. High attenuation in these masses causes shadowing of the deep portions of the liver.

B. These findings are confirmed on transverse scans which, again, show multiple echogenic metastases.

Echogenic metastases, in the author's experience, are rare in the untreated patient; when they occur, they are most frequently due to a mucin-secreting carcinoma of the colon. Mucin is a viscous substance which produces high-level echoes if seen in the gut or uterine cavity. It was therefore suggested that these appearances were due to hepatic metastases from an adenocarcinoma of the colon. Liver involve-ment was confirmed by isotope scanning, which showed multiple defects, while barium studies showed an apple-core carcinoma of the colon (Figure 4.19C).

This case demonstrates the value of ultrasound as an initial investigation of the patient with hepa-tomegaly. No other single, noninvasive investigation could provide the cause of the hepatic enlargement and an indication of the probable primary site of tumor. Echogenic metastases are, however, the exception rather than the rule, and even colonic tumors are frequently homogeneous. Some authors who report to the contrary show examples in which low gain setting and failure to display the normal parenchyma preclude the recognition of defects of the normal consistency. The format of a white image on a black background greatly facilitates the recognition of low echo-producing tumors.

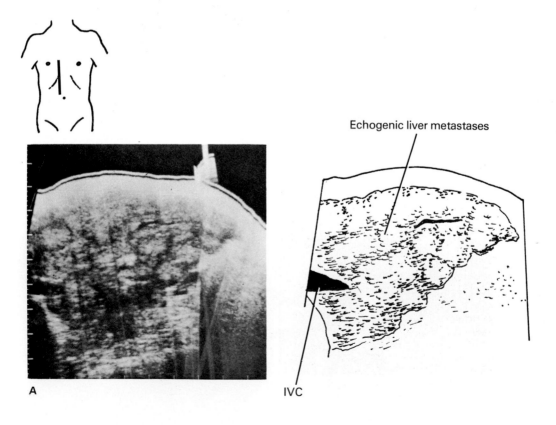

Echogenic liver metastases

A

IVC

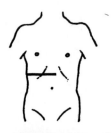

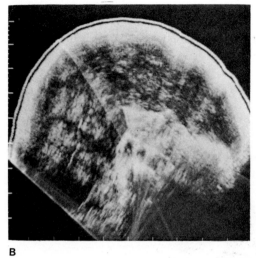

B

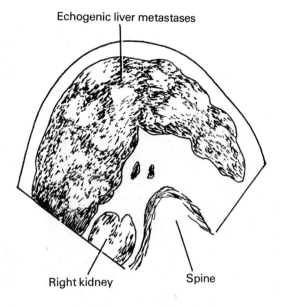

Echogenic liver metastases

Right kidney

Spine

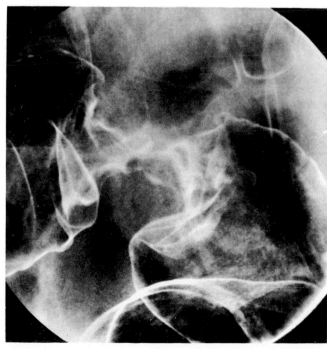

C

49

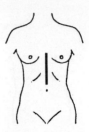

4.20 Malignancy—necrotic liver metastasis from carcinoma of the uterus

A 60-year-old female presented with a carcinoma of the body of the uterus. Ultrasound examination of the liver was carried out. A longitudinal section in the midline taken through the left lobe of the liver reveals a semifluid mass replacing the liver substance. Examination of the A-scan showed evidence of cellular debris, and the irregular walls suggested the possibility of a necrotic metastasis. This was confirmed at laparotomy.

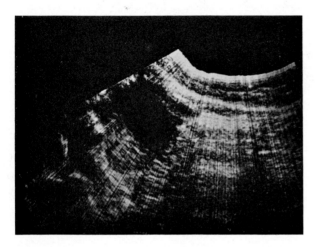

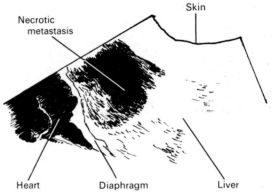

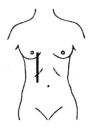

4.21 Malignancy—metastatic disease from islet cell tumor

This 55-year-old female presented with intractable jejunal ulceration and was found to have a pancreatic tumor causing the Zollinger–Ellison syndrome. At surgery large liver metastases were found and the patient was treated with chemotherapy for the subsequent three years. She was referred for ultrasound examination to evaluate the status of the liver involvement. This longitudinal ultrasonogram shows large cystic masses with smaller, solid components. These appearances are consistent with metastatic disease of the liver, which has been energetically treated.

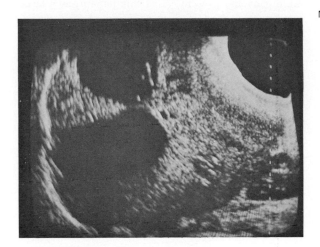
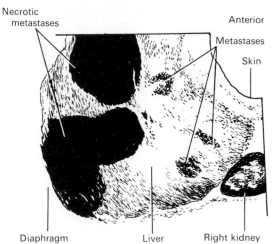

4.22 Malignancy—cystic metastases from ovarian cystadenocarcinoma

This 60-year-old woman presented with a palpable mass in the left hypochondrium which simulated splenomegaly. An ill-defined pelvic mass could be appreciated per abdomen. A paramedian ultrasonogram (upper figure) 2 cm to the left of the midline shows an entirely cystic mass with irregular contours, cellular debris, and evidence of local invasion into the liver. These appearances are obviously those of a malignant cyst and would be consistent with a secreting metastasis from a cystadenocarcinoma, of which the most common site of origin is the ovary.

Ultrasound examination of the pelvis (lower figure) in the midline shows a predominantly cystic mass lying posterior to the bladder, but superiorly there is a solid irregular component which suggests malignancy in this otherwise cystic ovarian mass. This was the primary ovarian cystadenocarcinoma.

Ovarian cystadenocarcinomata tend to form peritoneal metastases, which may later invade the underlying organs and present, as in this patient, as a large, cystic mass on the surface of the liver.

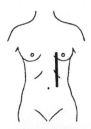

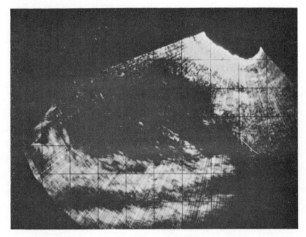

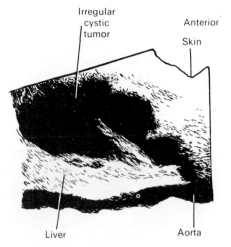

Irregular cystic tumor

Anterior

Skin

Liver

Aorta

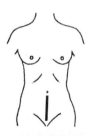

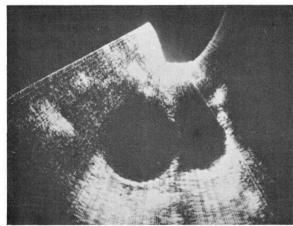

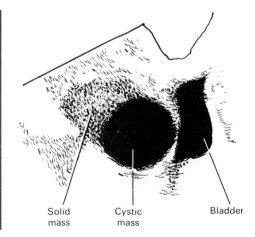

Solid mass

Cystic mass

Bladder

53

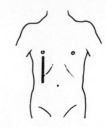

4.23 Malignancy—lymphoma

This 42-year-old patient with malignant lymphoma was referred for ultrasonic assessment of her liver. This parasagittal ultrasonogram through the right lobe of the liver shows three very homogeneous areas which display very low attenuation (note high echoes distal to lesions due to TGC through areas of low attenuation).

Lymphomas in liver may present as such highly homogeneous lesions as to simulate a cyst or an abscess. Unlike a cyst, there are very low-level echoes in the lymphoma lesion; this is best judged by inspection of the A-scan.

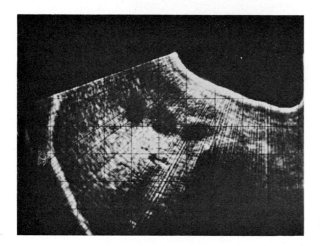

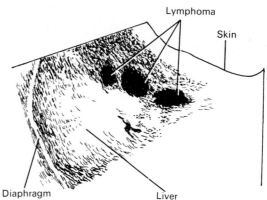

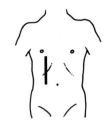

4.24 Malignancy—lymphoma

This 46-year-old male was known to suffer from a malignant lymphoma and was referred for ultrasound examination to assess the possibility of liver involvement. The paramedian ultrasound section through the right lobe of the liver and right kidney shows multiple defects, ranging in size from 2 mm to 2 cm. Such highly homogeneous tumors are characteristic of lymphomas, which make them easy to detect. As in this case, infiltrates as small as 2 to 3 mm are well delineated.

Chemotherapy may significantly alter these appearances and render them less well defined (see p. 57).

Gray scale ultrasound examination of the liver was evaluated for the staging of lymphomas prior to laparotomy. In 53 patients coming to a staging laparotomy, ultrasound correctly predicted liver involvement in 6 out of 8; and it correctly predicted noninvolvement in 42 out of 45.

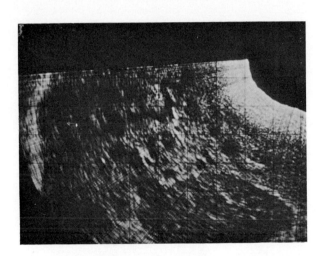

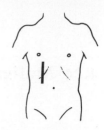

4.25 Malignancy—lymphoma and unsuccessful chemotherapy

A 28-year-old male absconded from a staging laparotomy for a malignant lymphoma and re-presented a year later with advanced disease in the thorax and para-aortic nodes. At that time, there was no evidence of liver involvement on ultrasonography. In view of his advanced disease, whole abdominal irradiation was carried out, sparing the upper half of the liver. The resulting liver changes showed diffuse high-level echoes, consistent with postirradiation fibrosis, while discrete, homogeneous (black) tumor deposits subsequently appeared in the liver. Clinically the patient deteriorated

rapidly and succumbed a week after the ultrasound scan shown here. The ultrasonogram is a paramedian section taken 6 cm to the right of the midline and shows an enlarged liver with high-level echoes interspersed by low-level tumor deposits. This interpretation was confirmed at postmortem. The right kidney can be seen posteriorly.

Abdominal irradiation in this patient was a last effort treatment, but in the presence of uncontrolled disease, it probably facilitated liver involvement by producing an arteritis in which malignant cells became trapped.

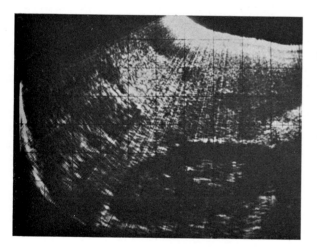

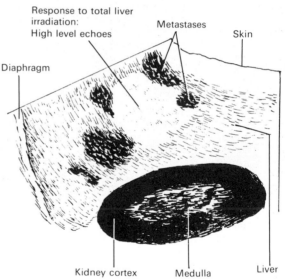

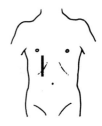

4.26 Malignancy—Hodgkin's disease successfully treated with chemotherapy

A 28-year-old male presented with widespread lymphadenopathy and hepatosplenomegaly. Lymphography demonstrated para-aortic lymphadenopathy and an inguinal node biopsy showed Hodgkin's disease. The paramedian ultrasonogram through the liver (upper figure) shows highly homogeneous areas which are characteristic of discrete Hodgkin's infiltration of the liver. This confirmed the clinical staging of 4B and chemotherapy was instituted. On clinical examination and lymphography, treatment produced an excellent response. A repeat ultrasonogram two months later shows disappearance of the previous abnormal areas and replacement by high echo areas, which attenuate the ultrasound beam and prevent display of the deeper tissues. Such appearances suggest fibrous replacement of tumor material. Experience showed that recurrence was heralded by reappearance of black areas shown in the upper figure.

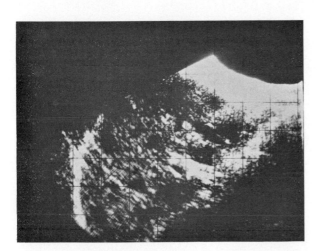

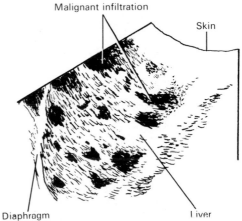

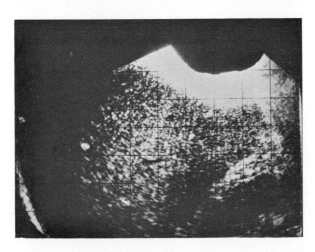

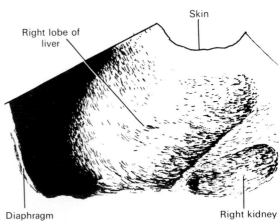

4.27 Malignancy—metastasis from oat cell carcinoma and failure of chemotherapy

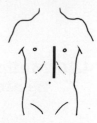

A 56-year-old male presented with hemoptyses and bronchoscopy revealed carcinoma of the bronchus, which proved on biopsy to be an "oat cell" carcinoma. He was referred for chemotherapy. On first presentation, liver ultrasonography revealed a definite homogeneous mass, interpreted as a metastasis on September 28. Chemotherapy was instituted and three months later the investigation was repeated (December 4). The metastasis had doubled in size despite treat-ment, the liver size had increased, and there were further areas of abnormality. The chemotherapeutic agents were changed, and a repeat ultrasonogram one month later (January 9) showed that the tumor growth had accelerated, so that the tumor areas had coalesced. The liver was now clinically malignantly involved. One month later (February 6), the tumor growth replaced all previous normal liver structure and the patient suc-cumbed.

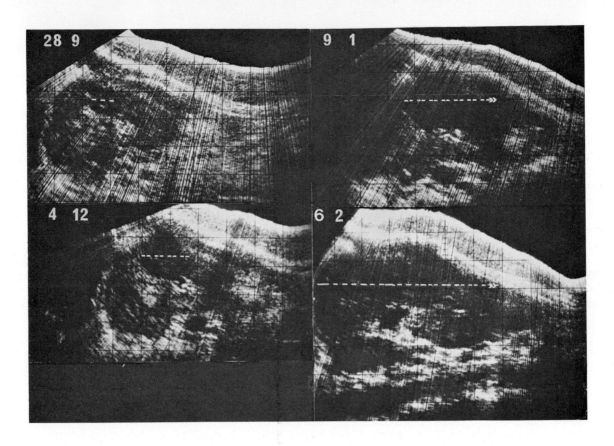

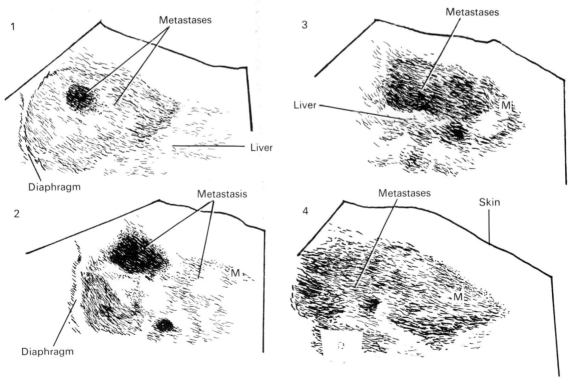

1

Metastases

Liver

Diaphragm

2

Metastasis

M

Diaphragm

3

Metastases

Liver

M

4

Metastases

Skin

M

59

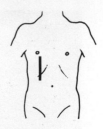

4.28 Malignancy—hemangioendothelioma

This 9-week-old infant was referred for ultrasonic investigation of the cause of hepatomegaly. A paramedian scan through the right lobe of the liver (upper figure) shows a homogeneous tumor 8 cm in diameter, producing echoes of lower amplitude than liver. The mass appears to be adjacent to, but not invading, the right kidney, which is just seen posteriorly.

A more medial section in the longitudinal plane of the inferior vena cava (middle figure) shows the tumor bulging into the lumen of the vena cava. Serial sections suggest marked vascularity. The appearances suggest a malignant tumor, although similar appearances may be mimicked by cavernous hemangiomata (see p. 35). At biopsy, the tumor was found to be highly vascular and bled profusely. The histology proved it to be a hemangioendothelioma.

Repeat examination after three weeks of steroid therapy shows a decrease in overall size and a change in consistency towards echoes of higher amplitude (lower figure). These appearances suggest tumor response to therapy.

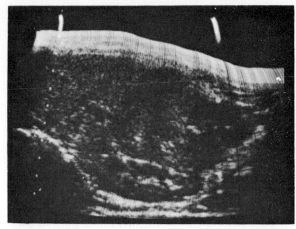

upper

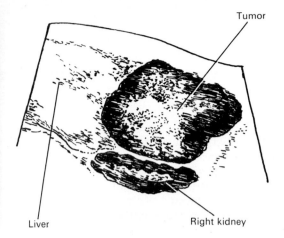

Tumor

Liver

Right kidney

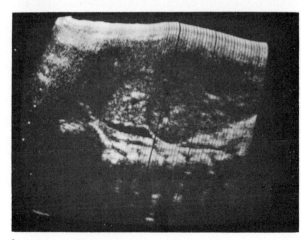

lower

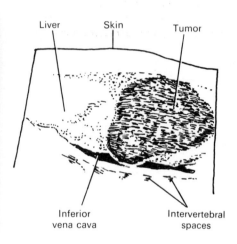

Liver   Skin   Tumor

Inferior
vena cava

Intervertebral
spaces

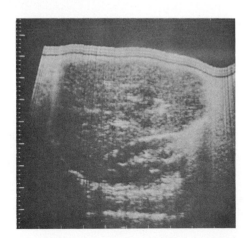

4.29 Primary tumor on chemotherapy

This 66-year-old patient with industrial exposure to chemicals developed a hemangiosarcoma of the liver, which was treated with intra-arterial adriamycin. Unfortunately, no baseline ultrasound examination was obtained before treatment.

This patient had multiple ultrasound examinations during treatment to estimate the size and consistency of the mass and, in particular, to look for signs of local spread. Over the course of one year, the appearances were remarkably stable, as was his clinical condition. The longitudinal ultrasonogram through the right lobe of the liver and right kidney (upper figure) shows a highly reflective mass 12 cm in diameter lying anterior

to the right kidney, while the transverse ultrasonogram (lower figure) shows a well-demarcated mass anterior to the right kidney and the great vessels. There appears to be extension on both sides of this mass. The appearances are those of a highly echogenic mass in the right lobe of the liver.

Sarcomatous tumors are usually highly homogeneous; it is therefore unfortunate that we do not have a baseline study on this patient before treatment. The appearances here of a tumor unchanging in size or consistency over the course of a year correlate extremely well with his clinical condition, which was stable.

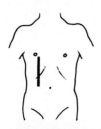

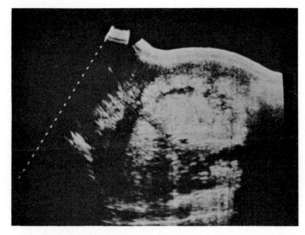

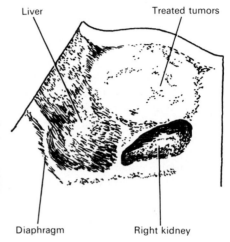

Liver

Treated tumors

Diaphragm

Right kidney

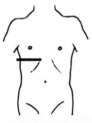

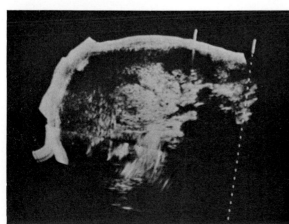

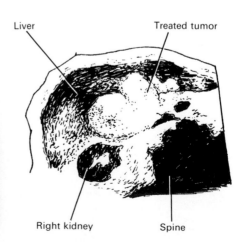

Liver

Treated tumor

Right kidney

Spine

4.30 Hepatoblastoma

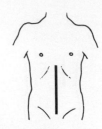

This 4-year-old boy presented with progressive increase in abdominal girth and was referred for ultrasonic evaluation of the abdomen before surgery. The ultrasonogram shown in the upper figure is a longitudinal section through the abdomen showing a thick rim of solid tumor in which the echoes are of irregular amplitude and the edges show irregularity; these findings are characteristic of malignant tumors. Posteriorly there is an echo-free space with low attenuation of irregular contour, and this is consistent with central necrosis occurring in the tumor. At surgery, these findings were confirmed, and the histology proved it to be a hepatoblastoma.

This child was treated with chemotherapy and local radiotherapy. Clinically the size of the tumor appeared to be increasing so that it appeared that there was no response to therapy. A repeat ultrasonogram (middle figure) showed that the increase in size was due to an increase in the central necrotic cavity and that the rim of solid tissue had in fact decreased in size. Note that there are more high-level echoes also present in this tumor material. On this evidence from the ultrasonic examination, a needle was placed into the abdomen but no fluid was obtained. The procedure was repeated after ultrasound localization of optimal needle site. On this occasion, 1200 ml of serosanguineous fluid were aspirated.

Repeated ultrasound examination (lower figure) at the end of radiotherapy showed that the abdominal cavity was largely filled with a necrotic cystic area with irregular strands of residual tumor. Repeat aspiration was required. Subsequently this tumor slowly recurred despite continuing chemotherapy and showed progressive replacement of the cystic areas with more solid components until the child succumbed.

This case illustrates the clinical importance of the ability to differentiate solid from cystic masses in the management of the patient. In this child, it appeared from clinical examination that this tumor was unresponsive to the therapy, whereas ultrasonic examination clearly revealed a decrease in the solid tumor component. This case also demonstrates the use of ultrasound to guide the surgeon to the optimal site for needle aspiration, now a routine application for ultrasound but a new application at the time that this child was scanned.

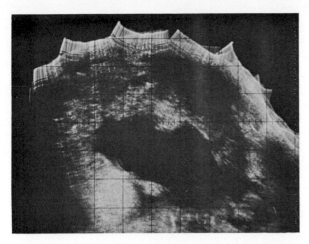
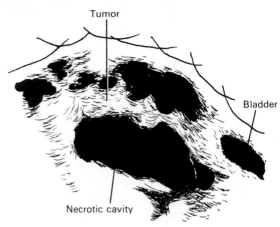

Tumor

Bladder

Necrotic cavity

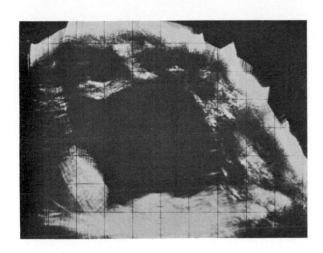

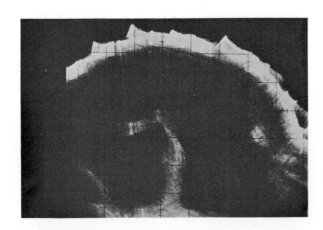

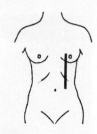

4.31 Benign tumor—adenoma

This 22-year-old female had been using contraceptive pills for two years. She was referred for ultrasound when hepatomegaly was noted on routine physical examination. Liver biopsy revealed peliosis hepatis. Angiography showed a vascular mass occupying the left lobe of the liver. Ultrasound reveals a highly reflective tumor in the left lobe of the liver. The mass appears to be well circumscribed and uniform throughout. At surgery, an adenoma was found.

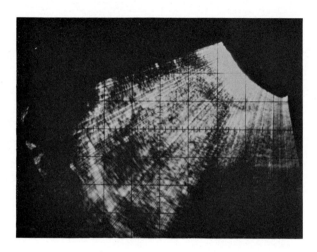

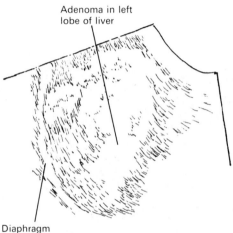

Adenoma in left lobe of liver

Diaphragm

4.32 Renal cell carcinoma simulating primary liver tumor

This 23-year-old patient presented to the emergency room with a history of an increasing mass in the right upper quadrant of six weeks' duration. Soon after admission the mass became acutely painful and she became hypotensive. Emergency examination was requested to assess the nature of the patient's upper abdominal pathology.

Three longitudinal ultrasound sections are seen (A, B and C) through the upper abdomen at relatively low gain. The transverse ultrasonogram (D) is shown. Liver tissue is seen anteriorly on all sections, while occupying the usual position of the liver is a large, highly reflective mass. There is evidence of large feeding vessels and more irregular areas which are echo-free with irregular contours, and these suggest areas of necrosis and frank hemorrhage into a tumor. All these appearances are consistent with a highly vascular tumor replacing most of the liver substance. At this stage it appeared that this

was most probably a primary liver tumor, since these appearances are highly unusual for untreated metastatic disease. Examination did, however, provide an immediate answer as to the nature of the mass in an emergency situation.

The following morning a liver-spleen scan was performed with 99 m Technetium labeled sulphur colloid. This scan suggests the presence of a tumor compressing the liver from its posterior aspect, but certainly does not give the impression of the very large size of the tumor that is apparent from the ultrasonograms. Angiography revealed a tumor the size of a football arising from the right kidney, with malignant extensions into the renal vein and inferior vena cava. The patient died of a saddle embolus during the course of attempted removal of the tumor. Histology revealed a clear cell carcinoma.

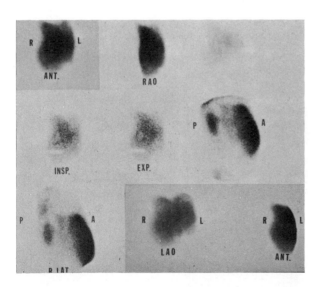

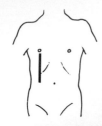

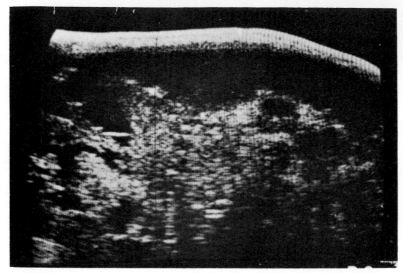

A

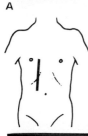

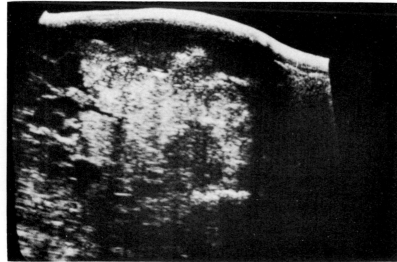

B

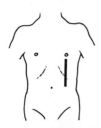

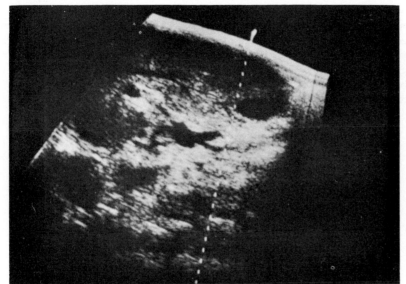

C

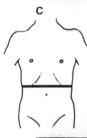

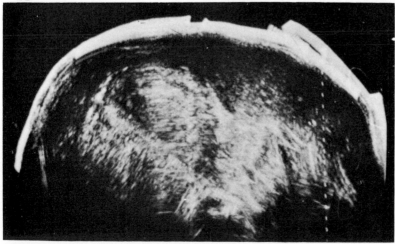

D

4.33 Metabolic changes—fatty infiltration

A 40-year-old female with a 10 year history of malignant hypertension presented in hepatorenal failure. She was referred for ultrasound examination of the liver.

A longitudinal ultrasonogram (upper figure) showed marked enlargement of the liver with high-level echoes distributed in a fine pattern but with normal attenuation. Obvious vessels are frequently seen. The gallbladder is demonstrated and is normal in size.

A transverse ultrasonogram (lower figure) confirms the abnormal liver consistency, which is characteristic of fatty infiltration. Note that the stomach can be seen on this ultrasonogram as a fluid containing viscus with a corrugated wall.

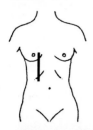

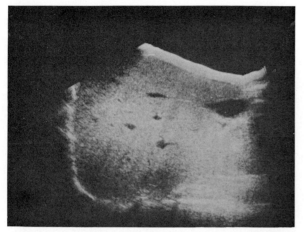

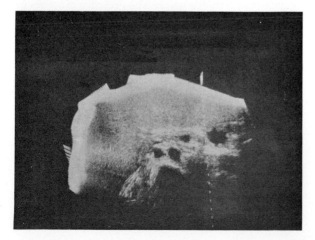

4.34 Metabolic changes—cirrhosis of the liver

This middle-aged man presented with jaundice and a long history of alcohol abuse. Obvious ascites was apparent. He was referred for ultrasound examination to exclude extrahepatic cause for his jaundice, which might be amenable to surgical relief.

A parasagittal ultrasonogram (upper figure) through the right lobe of the liver and right kidney shows the liver to be surrounded by ascites both on its anterior aspect and between the visceral surface of the liver and right kidney (Morison's pouch). On the anterior surface of the liver, the lumen of the gallbladder is barely seen. The liver itself displays a highly abnormal consistency with dense white echoes and inadequate penetration to the deep surface. This suggests that there is both an increase in the echoes from the liver and increased attenuation within the liver. These findings are diagnostic of diffuse intrahepatic fibrosis and consistent with cirrhosis. There is no evidence of biliary tree dilatation.

The lower figure shows a small sector scan through the ascites and displays the right kidney in cross section. The increased gain produced by the beam passing through the ascites and receiving TGC without attenuation by the ascitic fluid demonstrates more structure within the kidney than is usually apparent. In this patient the pyramids are clearly demarcated, allowing discrimination between the cortex and medulla.

This case demonstrates the characteristic findings in cirrhosis, to which may be added the appearances of the portal vein and congestive splenomegaly (Fig. 4.36). Computerized A-scan analysis by Mountford and Wells (1972) has quantitatively proved that larger echoes emanate from cirrhotic livers than from normal livers. The increased attenuation from cirrhotic livers enables this entity to be differentiated from purely fatty infiltration. In our experience to date, it appears that regenerative nodules do not appear ultrasonically different from the surrounding tissue, so that any evidence of a homogeneous tumor must be regarded as a possible malignancy. Such cases clearly show the advantage of ultrasound over CT in the investigation of the liver, since the liver consistency is so well demonstrated by ultrasound without the use of contrast media and specific changes are seen with increasing intrahepatic fibrosis due to the dependence of echo amplitude on collagen interfaces (see p. 7).

This case also demonstrates the use of ultrasound to diagnose differentially obstructive jaundice and, in particular, to determine whether it is due to extrahepatic or intrahepatic causes. The inability in this patient to display any evidence of a dilated biliary tree suggests that the liver failure is due to intrinsic disease. Not infrequently, patients present with a mixture of intrinsic and extrinsic causes for jaundice which must be differentiated. Patients with cirrhosis or malignant infiltration of the liver may present with jaundice apparently due to intrinsic liver disease; but ultrasound demonstrates dilated ducts in addition, suggesting that at least part of their jaundice is due to extrahepatic compression by involved lymph nodes, incidental gallstones, etc. The ability to distinguish dilated biliary ducts—which is achieved at this center with an accuracy of 96.7%—allows one to recognize any extrahepatic obstruction and perform palliative surgery.

Although it has recently been suggested that ascites is never seen in the hepatorenal angle, this is totally contrary to our experience and, as in this case, ascites is frequently seen in this space. The presence of ascites in this patient allowed us to visualize the pyramids with clarity for the first time. With improved instrumentation, these are now displayed in 50% of our patients in routine examination.

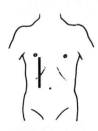

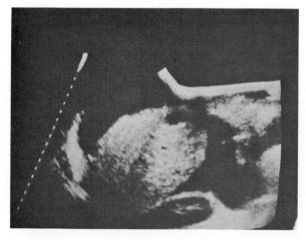

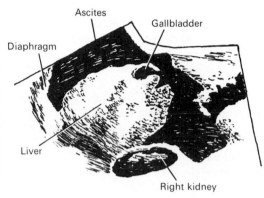

Ascites

Gallbladder

Diaphragm

Liver

Right kidney

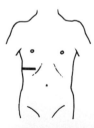

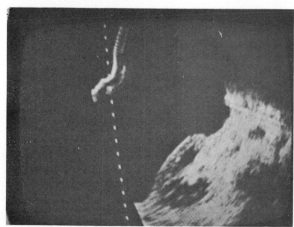

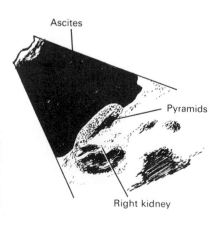

Ascites

Pyramids

Right kidney

4.35 Metabolic changes—severe cirrhosis of the liver

Cirrhosis is characterized by the progressive replacement of the liver parenchyma by fibrous scar tissue and, since collagen appears to be a major site for echo formation, more echoes may be expected from the increased collagen content. Quantitative A-scan analysis has confirmed an increased amplitude of echoes from cirrhotic liver (Mountford and Wells, 1972). Thus the A-scan through the cirrhotic liver shows high-level echoes from within the liver of similar size to that from the diaphragm. In the normal A-scan, the intrahepatic echoes are only half to one-third the size of the diaphragmatic echo.

However, in severe cirrhosis the ultrasound beam is rapidly attenuated so that little energy reaches the deeper tissues; therefore, only small echoes are returned from them. Thus, in the severe cirrhotic, very high-level echoes are seen superficially but high attenuation reduces the amplitude of the deeper echoes (upper figure). On the B-scan, this results in dense high-level echoes from the superficial tissues but a failure to display the deeper parts of the liver. Usually, the diaphragm is barely seen (lower figure).

The TGC can be manipulated to improve the quality of the image; for example, the near gain can be reduced and the overall gain increased. This change of TGC is necessary to correct the abnormally high attenuation, and this must be recalled in the interpretation of the scan. Ideally, a quantitative measure of tissue attenuation should be made.

When severe cirrhosis prevents penetration to the deep portions of the liver, a frequency of 1.6 MHz can be used; but again, it must be recalled that this is necessary only because of the abnormally high attenuation by the liver that is characteristic of cirrhosis. Other pathology—such as fatty infiltration, which gives high-level echoes—does not produce a significant increase in attenuation. The changes seen in cirrhosis are simulated by any other pathology which results in diffuse intrahepatic fibrosis, e.g. congenital hepatic fibrosis (p. 39).

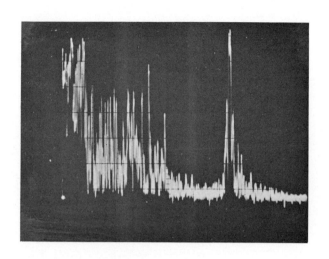

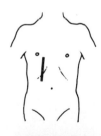

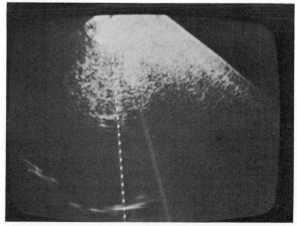

4.36 Metabolic changes—cirrhosis of liver producing portal hypertension and congestive splenomegaly

This 61-year-old male presented with hepatomegaly and jaundice. He was referred for ultrasonic examination to elucidate the cause of his liver failure. A paramedian scan through the liver substance 2 cm to the right of the midline (upper figure) shows a diffusely abnormal liver consistency with high-level echoes, but of note is a large, highly tortuous portal vein. This strongly suggests portal hypertension. Splenic exam-ination in the decubitus position reveals marked splenomegaly (lower figure). The longitudinal axis of the spleen measures 18 cm (normal, less than 10 cm). There are medium-level echoes returned evenly throughout the organ and these appearances are consistent with congestive splenomegaly associated with portal hypertension due to cirrhosis. A barium swallow demonstrated marked esophageal varices.

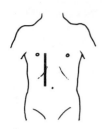

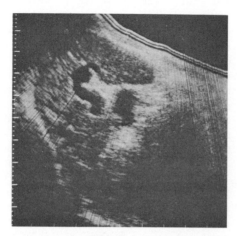

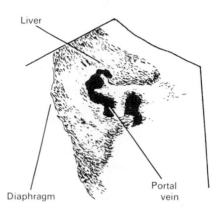

Liver

Diaphragm

Portal vein

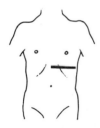

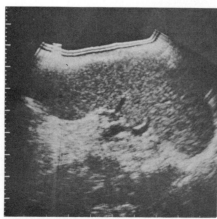

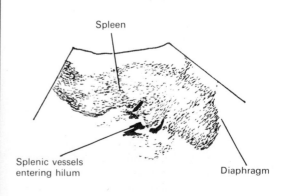

Spleen

Splenic vessels entering hilum

Diaphragm

RELATION OF ULTRASOUND TO OTHER MODALITIES FOR IMAGING THE LIVER

K.J.W. Taylor and D. Sullivan

Isotope liver scanning has been widely used to image the liver for the past 15 years. The method involves isotopic labeling of a colloid. The colloid is phagocytosed by the Kupffer's cells, which permits the liver to be imaged on a gamma camera. Thus the imaging process depends upon the physiological function of the liver, which may be impaired by cytotoxic agents. Numerous reports claim an accuracy of between 72% and 90% (Baum, Silver, Vouchides, 1966; Czerniak, 1964; Drum and Christacopoulis, 1972; Gollin, Sims, and Cameron, 1964; McAfee, Ause, and Wagner, 1965; Nagler, Bender, and Blau, 1963). The introduction of Technetium, which is a rather ideal pharmaceutical, did not substantially improve the accuracy rates; nor have increasingly sophisticated gamma cameras now using 37 photomultiplier tubes substantially improved the results of the examination. In a recent study, defects in the porta hepatis were found to represent significant pathology in 42% of the population and anatomical variation in 58% (McClelland, 1975). Such equivocal results are of little use in the clinical management of the patient.

A prospective study of 95 patients was undertaken on whom equivocal results of the isotopic liver scans were found between July 1, 1976 and February 1, 1977. All isotopic examinations were carried out on a state of the art, 37 photomultiplier tube camera; and all patients received a gray scale ultrasonographic examination within two days of the isotope scan, and usually within one hour. Of the 90 proven follow-ups to date, the overall accuracy for ultrasonic examination was 94%. This accuracy increased to 96% when both examinations were considered together. An analysis of some of the subgroups showed that, in the presence of an equivocal liver scan, when the ultrasound was normal the liver was normal with a high reliability of 89% in this series. Furthermore, when the liver scintigram was equivocal but probably abnormal and the ultrasound was definitely abnormal, the liver was abnormal in 100% in this series.

Although we have occasionally, during the past four years, encountered significant pathology on the ultrasound liver scan in the presence of a normal isotope scan, this is unusual; thus the isotope liver scan can be used as a screening procedure in the initial investigation of the liver. Equivocal isotope scans should be further investigated either by ultrasound or by CT scanning. There are strong proponents for either technique, and the favored method should obviously be the technique which produces the highest accuracy rate most economi-

cally. Since, in the study reported here, the combination of ultrasound and isotope scanning of the liver resulted in accuracy of 96%, few cases need to be investigated by more invasive or expensive methods.

In the investigation of a definitely positive nuclear scan, ultrasound or CT scanning can be used to differentially diagnose the cause of space-occupying lesions and, in particular, to differentiate between solid and cystic composition. Again, ultrasound presents itself as a highly accurate method which permits this differentiation most economically. One important advantage of ultrasound over CT scanning is the ability to display the normal consistency of the liver without the use of contrast media. The difference between the X-ray absorption of normal tissue and cirrhotic liver tissue is not large enough to allow discrimination by CT; yet this can eaily be achieved by ultrasonic visualization. For the accurate recognition of metastatic disease of the liver, contrast media are required for CT scanning while, again, this is not necessary for ultrasound scanning. Thus it appears that ultrasound, both because of the high resolution and good tissue differentiation, is the most valuable method for further investigating the cause of equivocal and positive isotope liver scans. In a small number of patients, further investigation by CT or more invasive methods may be necessary. Some case histories are now presented which show the practical value of ultrasound in the interpretation of potential liver pathology as identified by the isotope liver scan (Figs. 4.37–4.46).

We have also investigated the combined use of ultrasound and ^{67}Gallium scans for the diagnosis of abdominal abscesses. Gallium uptake is nonspecific and is found in inflammatory, neoplastic, or traumatic lesions. However, when a fluid collection is demonstrated by ultrasound and is shown to take up Gallium, there is strong evidence for an abscess cavity. The combination of the two techniques reduces the incidence of false positives by either examination when performed alone. This is demonstrated in Figures 4.47 and 4.48, in which positive Gallium uptake in the liver is shown by ultrasound to be either an abscess or a diffuse inflammation due to sarcoidosis.

REFERENCES

Baum, S., Silver, J., and Vouchides, D.: The recognition of hepatic metastases through radioisotope colour scanning. *J. Am. Med. Assoc.*, **197**, 675–679, 1966.

Czerniak, P.: Scanning study of 700 livers: evaluation of existing diagnostic procedures. In *Medical Radioisotope Scanning*, Vol. 2, International Atomic Energy Agency, Vienna, 1964, pp. 401–424.

Drum, D.E. and Christacopoulis, J.S.: Hepatic scintigraphy in clinical decision making. *J. Nucl. Med.*, **13**, 908–915, 1972.

Gollin, F.F., Sims, J.L., and Cameron, J.R.: Liver scanning and liver function tests. *J. Am. Med. Assoc.*, **187,** 111–116, 1964

McAfee, I.G., Ause, R.G. and Wagner, H.N.: Diagnostic value of scintillation scanning of the liver. *Arch. Intern. Med.*, **116,** 95–110, 1965.

Nagler, W., Bender, M.A., and Blau, M: Radioisotope photoscanning of the liver. *Gastroenterol.*, **44,** 36–43, 1963.

McClelland, R.R.: Focal portahepatis scintiscan defects: what is their significance? *J. Nucl. Med.*, **16,** 1007–1012, 1975.

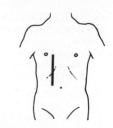

4.37 Positive isotope scan differentiated by ultrasound liver scan. Inflammatory state —chronic active hepatitis

This 37-year-old male was referred for examination because of repeated attacks of upper abdominal pain and transient jaundice. A 99 m Technetium sulphur colloid isotope scan (above) reveals a defect in the right lobe of the liver, while the ultrasound scan (below) permits further differentiation. The longitudinal scan shows a dense mass of high-level echoes from within the liver substance which is consistent with a chronic in-flammatory process. At biopsy, chronic active hepatitis was diagnosed. In addition, despite prolonged fasting, the gallbladder lumen was not visualized in this patient and there was no evidence of any shadowing or suggestion of gallstones. This suggested that this patient might have a small contracted gallbladder which was incapable of physiological distention. At surgery, a small contracted gallbladder without gallstones was found.

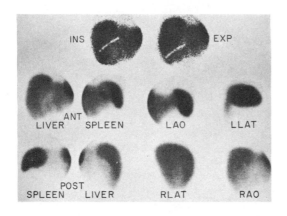

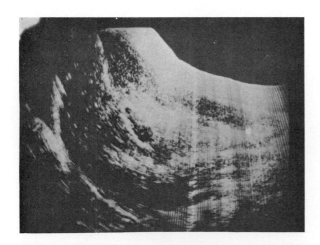

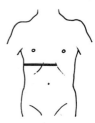

4.38 Positive isotope scan differentiated by ultrasound

A 60-year-old patient was referred for investigation after primary treatment for a melanoma. The isotope liver scan showed a defect in the posterior aspect of the liver and, in addition, there was more uptake in the left lobe of the liver than in the right. Metastatic disease in the posterior of the right lobe was suggested by these appearances. He was referred for ultrasound to confirm this possibility.

The transverse ultrasonogram reveals a large, predominantly acoustically homogeneous tumor extending into the liver tissue from the posterior aspect; smaller satellite tumors are clearly defined. The appearances are consistent with metastatic melanoma.

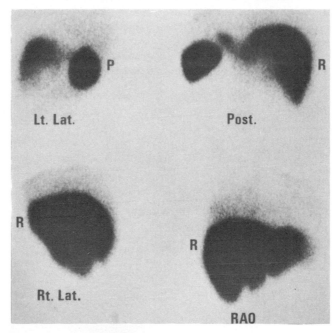

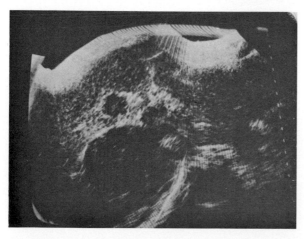

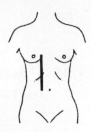

4.39 Positive isotope scan differentiated by ultrasound

This 50-year-old woman, who had a carcinoma of the breast treated by a radical mastectomy, presented for routine examination and was referred for isotope evaluation of the liver.

The isotope liver examination shows a large cold area in the region of the porta hepatis and extending out into the right lobe of the liver. Clinically, however, this patient did not appear to have metastatic disease and there was no evidence of abnormal liver function. In view of this apparent conflict between the results of the isotope examination and the clinical impression, she was referred for ultrasonic evaluation of the liver.

A longitudinal ultrasound section through the right lobe of the liver reveals a large echo-free area. the A-scan through the lesion was completely flat, and there was no evidence of attenuation within the lesion. The walls are regular and the appearances are those of a simple cyst, probably of congenital origin. There is no evidence of tumor involvement of the liver.

Incidental liver cysts may produce great concern when they produce a space-occupying defect on the isotope scan and simulate metastatic involvement. Immediate ultrasound examination in these patients relieves the patients' minds and resolves the clinician's dilemma of whether to institute dangerous treatment based on the isotope scan.

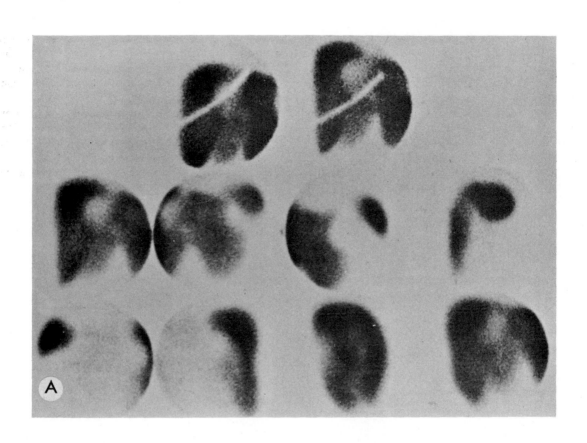

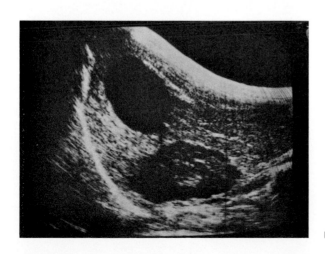

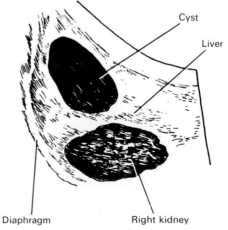

Cyst

Liver

Diaphragm

Right kidney

4.40 Positive isotope scan differentiated by ultrasound scan

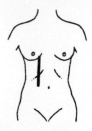

This 14-year-old girl presented with a pelvic mass, which proved to be a malignant teratoma (p. 358). This was excised and she was given chemotherapy. Subsequently, she was referred for isotope and ultrasound liver scans in a search for metastatic disease. Three months after her original surgery, a defect was noted on the upper border of the right lobe of the liver; these appearances were consistent with either a tumor replacing the upper part of the right lobe of the liver or a subphrenic abscess. She was referred for ultrasonic examination to differentiate between these possibilities.

A longitudinal parasagittal ultrasonogram through the right lobe of the liver shows a highly reflective mass on the superior aspect of the liver. In patients who are undergoing chemotherapy, such appearances are consistent with metastatic disease.

These appearances were confirmed at angiography, which showed a mass which was fed by branches of the phrenic arteries and appeared to be a peritoneal deposit compressing the liver substance. At surgery a large peritoneal metastasis was excised, and the patient remains well 10 months after this surgery.

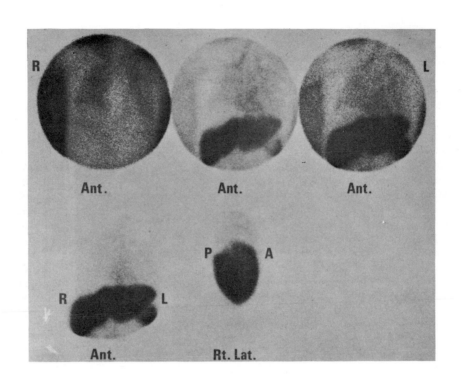

R   Ant.   Ant.   Ant.   L

P   A

R   L

Ant.   Rt. Lat.

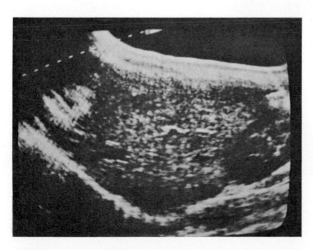

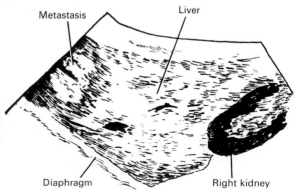

Metastasis   Liver

Diaphragm   Right kidney

4.41 Equivocal isotope liver scan differentiated by ultrasound

This 29-year-old woman who was an alcoholic presented with signs of advanced liver failure, including jaundice. She was referred for an isotopic liver-spleen scan.

An anterior view of the liver-spleen scan shows an enlarged liver with patchy uptake of isotope and a definite cold area in the region of the porta hepatis extending into the right lobe. The spleen is moderately enlarged with good uptake of isotope. There is marked uptake of isotope in the bone marrow of the ribs, sternum, and vertebral bodies, indicating severe liver damage. These appearances are consistent with cirrhosis, but also raise the question of the nature of the cold area in the porta hepatis and extending into the right lobe. The possibility of malignant transformation in this area cannot be excluded. Because of this equivocal result, she was referred for ultrasonic evaluation of the liver.

A transverse ultrasonogram (upper figure) shows that the liver consistency is abnormal, and there are dense white echoes returned from the liver substance. The use

of a compound scanning technique masks any increase in attenuation. Attention is directed towards the region of the porta hepatis, in which a cystic structure can be seen, which is clearly the gallbladder. Note that there is also a fluid interval between the liver and the anterior abdominal wall, and a further interval between the liver and lateral border of the right kidney. This is consistent with a small quantity of ascitic fluid.

A longitudinal ultrasonogram (lower figure) confirms the presence of the gallbladder in a medial position and lying immediately anterior to the inferior vena cava.

The ultrasound appearances seen here of dense white echoes originating from the liver substance with ascites are part of the spectrum of changes seen in cirrhosis of the liver. The gallbladder in this patient is unusually medially placed, but there are marked variations in the anatomical position of the gallbladder, which indeed may be on a mesentery and therefore freely mobile. On the basis of the ultrasound scans, it was possible to exclude malignant transformation in the cold area noted on the nuclear scan.

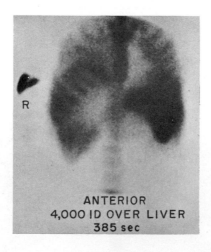

ANTERIOR
4,000 ID OVER LIVER
385 sec

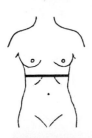

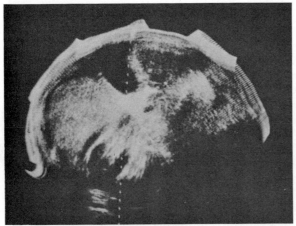

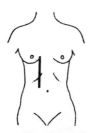

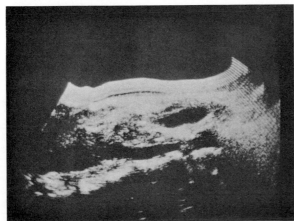

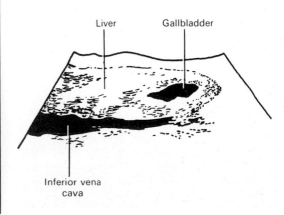

Liver   Gallbladder

Inferior vena
cava

87

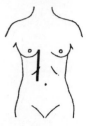

4.42 Equivocal nuclear scan differentiated by ultrasound

This 55-year-old patient was referred for evaluation of the liver because of a known carcinoma of the ovary.

The isotope liver scan shows a definite defect in the interlobar fissure, which may occur either as an anatomical variant or may represent significant pathology. She was referred for ultrasound evaluation in view of this equivocal result.

The longitudinal ultrasonogram shows the region of the porta hepatis. A large homogeneous tumor is seen which has irregular edges, strongly suggesting local invasion. The appearances are therefore of a metastatic lesion 7.5 cm in diameter.

Despite therapy, this patient rapidly deteriorated and succumbed to metastatic disease of the liver. The equivocal isotope results, compared with the large size of this tumor apparent on the ultrasound examination, provide an indication of the relative insensitivity of the isotope examination.

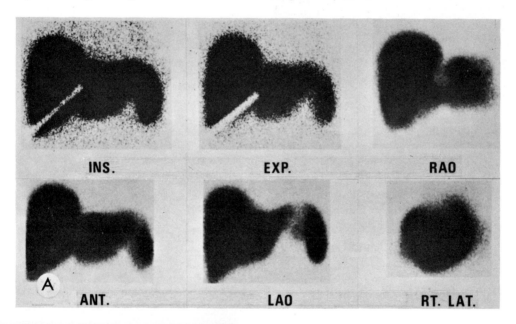

INS.   EXP.   RAO

ANT.   LAO   RT. LAT.

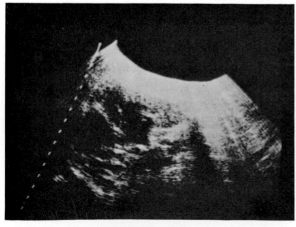

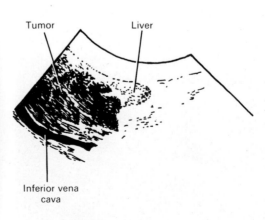

Tumor   Liver

Inferior vena cava

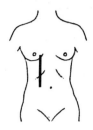

4.43 Equivocal isotope scan differentiated by ultrasound

This 50-year-old female had a ductal carcinoma of the breast and was referred for a liver scan as part of her routine follow-up.

The isotope liver scan shows thinning of the inferior edge of the right lobe of the liver. Since the presence of small space-occupying lesions could not be excluded, the patient was referred for ultrasonic evaluation of the liver.

Ultrasound examination reveals a liver of a normal consistency, although the right lobe of the liver is thin and extends anteriorly as a Riedel's lobe.

A clinical follow-up 12 months after these scans were taken shows no evidence of metastatic disease or further deterioration of the isotope liver scan. It was concluded that these appearances were due to anatomical variation and not metastatic disease.

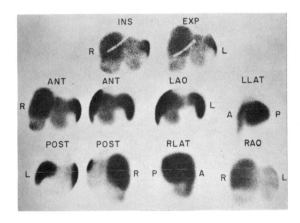

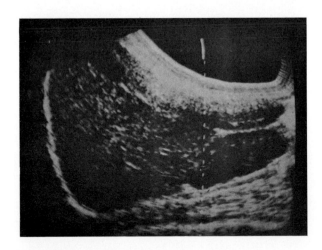

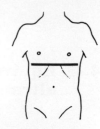

4.44 Equivocal isotope scan differentiated by ultrasound

A 60-year-old male presented with ascites of one week's duration and hiccuping. The possibility of a sub-diaphragmatic abscess was considered, and the patient was referred for isotope examination.

Isotope examination revealed a small liver with decreased and patchy uptake. Since focal defects could not be excluded because of patchy uptake, ultrasound was suggested. There was shift of colloid to the spleen, which was massively enlarged.

Transverse ultrasonic examination reveals high-level echoes throughout the liver substance with marked ascites around the liver. The spleen is enlarged. There is no evidence of any tumor. The appearances are those of cirrhosis, with splenomegaly and ascites. On neither isotope nor ultrasound scan was a subphrenic abscess apparent.

This patient proved to have cardiac cirrhosis due to congestive cardiac failure with ascites, but no evidence of a subphrenic abscess was found.

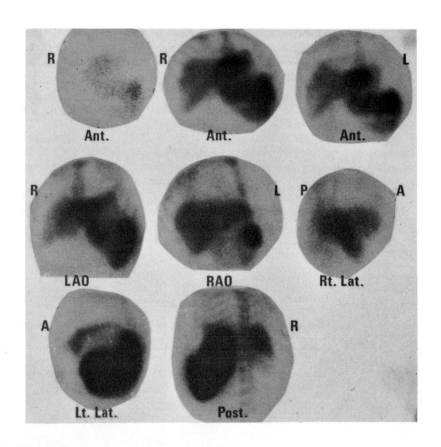

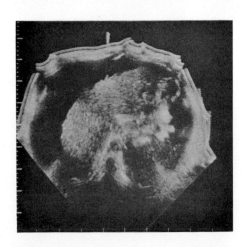

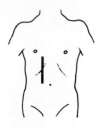

4.45 Equivocal isotope scan differentiated by ultrasound

In a 76-year-old patient who presented with obstructive jaundice, hepatomegaly was noted on clinical examination. Pronounced weight loss had occurred. The patient was referred for isotopic evaluation of the liver to exclude metastatic disease.

The isotope scan confirms hepatomegaly, and a lobulated appearance is noted. There is non-homogeneous distribution of activity with a cold area in the region of the porta hepatis, which could be due to dilated ducts or enlarged nodes. There is a shift of colloid to the spleen.

Multiple sections through the liver on ultrasonic examination failed to reveal evidence of metastatic disease, although there is definite dilatation of the biliary tree with distention of the cystic duct and the gallbladder contains sludge. The appearances were those of obstruction to the common bile duct due to an unknown cause, producing biliary dilatation but no evidence of liver metastases.

At surgery a carcinoma of the pancreas was found. There was biliary dilatation but no evidence of metastasis either to the nodes or to the liver. This case is a typical example of the use of ultrasound to diagnose extrahepatic biliary obstruction, but the precise site of the obstruction may be more difficult to locate accurately due to air in the overlying gut.

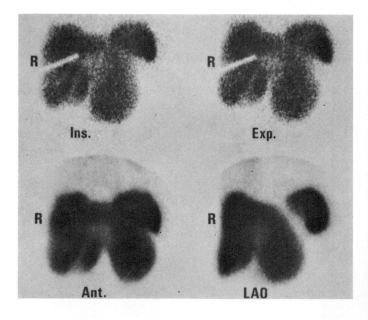

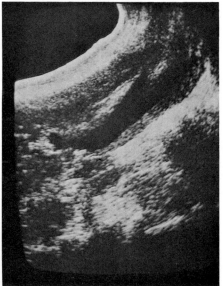

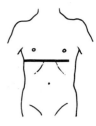

4.46 Equivocal isotope scan differentiated by ultrasound

A 66-year-old patient presented with congestive cardiac failure, recent increase in liver size, and abnormal liver function tests.

The isotope liver scan shows hepatomegaly with uneven activity. There are defects in the right lobe to the right of the spine which are seen in the posterior view. The right lateral view suggests two further filling defects. Ultrasound was suggested to differentiate the possible cause of these defects.

The ultrasound examination revealed hepatomegaly; on this transverse section, gross dilatation of the hepatic veins and inferior vena cava can be seen. These vessels are sufficiently large to produce significant filling defects on the isotope scan. No evidence of any further space-occupying lesions was found.

Follow-up confirmed that the liver changes were secondary to congestive cardiac failure and there was no evidence of any tumor.

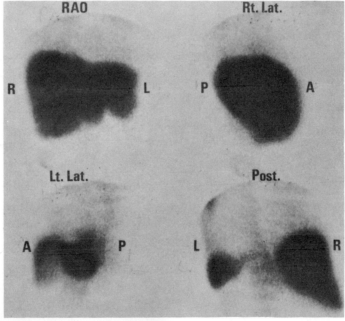

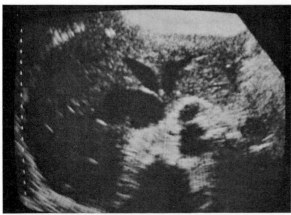

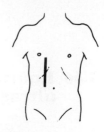

4.47 Positive ^{67}Gallium scan differentiated by ultrasound

A 40-year-old patient presented with a one month history of intermittent right upper quadrant pain and fever. A ^{99m}Technetium sulphur colloid liver scan showed a defect in the right lobe. Ultrasound examination reveals a large abnormality which consists of a thick rim of high-level echoes with low central ones. These appearances are characteristic of a thick fibrous capsule surrounding an abscess cavity and, in the experience of the author, are diagnostic of a liver abscess. A Gallium scan shows uptake in the area in question. The blood cultures were positive for *Staph. aureus* and subsequent surgical draining confirmed a pyogenic abscess.

In our experience with ultrasound and Gallium scans, the combination of ^{67}Gallium uptake in an area shown to be a fluid collection by ultrasound is very strong evidence for the presence of an abscess.

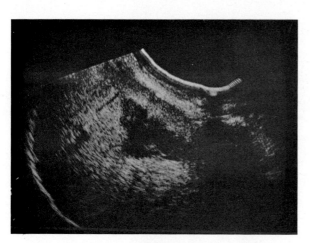

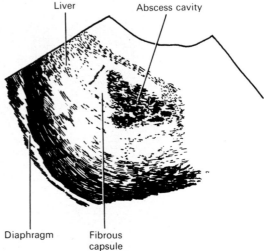

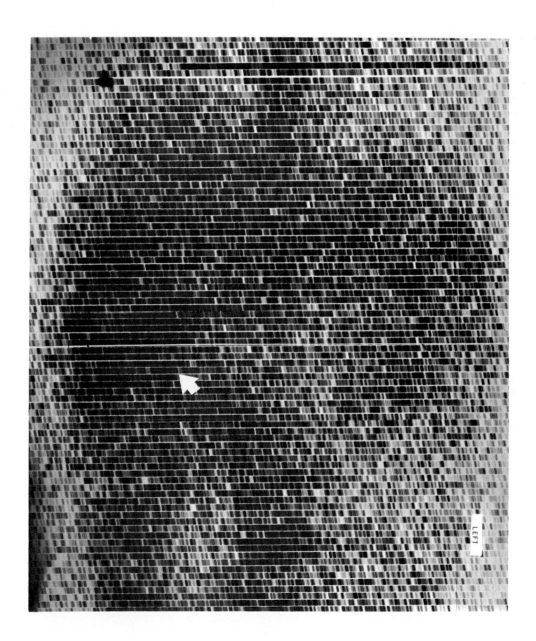

4.48 Positive Gallium scan differentiated by ultrasound

This is a 36-year-old female who presented with massive hepatomegaly on clinical examination. A Technetium sulphur colloid isotopic scan (A) shows marked enlargement of the liver with several defects. A Gallium scan (B) shows that the focal lesions on the Technetium scan concentrate [67]Gallium, demonstrating functional activity in these areas which is either inflammatory or neoplastic in nature.

A longitudinal ultrasonogram (C) shows a markedly abnormal liver consistency with diffuse high-level echoes consistent with a diffuse inflammatory granulomatous reaction in the liver without evidence of abscess formation.

The ultrasound examination differentiated first between a tumor and an inflammatory process and, furthermore, excluded the presence of an abscess cavity. Histological examination showed sarcoidosis.

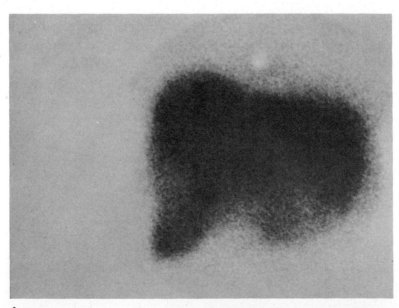

A

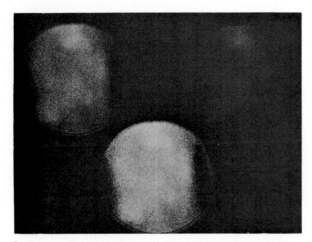

B

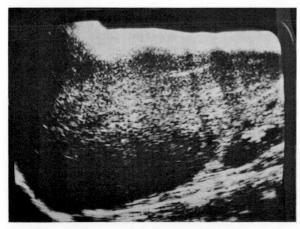

C

97

5. The biliary system

5.1 Normal anatomy of the gallbladder

Patients are fasted for at least eight hours before gallbladder examination to produce physiological distention of the gallbladder. A paramedian scan through the right lobe of the liver (upper figure) shows the gallbladder, pyriform in contour, usually situated on the inferior (visceral) surface of the liver. Wide variations occur in the size, shape, and position of the gallbladder. The gallbladder may be embedded in the liver, producing an intrahepatic gallbladder, or it may be suspended on a mesentery. The size of the gallbladder shows wide variations in length, which may be up to 12 cm. Conversely, many obstructed gallbladders may be less than 12 cm long. Even when the anterior approach to the gallbladder is difficult due to air in the colon, the gallbladder fossa can always be imaged by sector scans through the intercostal spaces (p. 21).

An oblique ultrasonogram (lower figure) along the line of the costal margin shows the lumen of the gallbladder converging into the cystic duct. Note the spiral valve arrangement in the neck of the gallbladder.

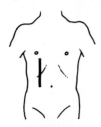

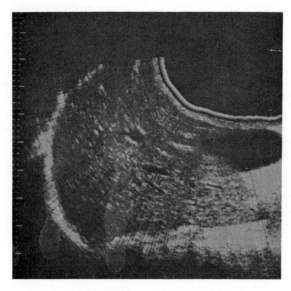

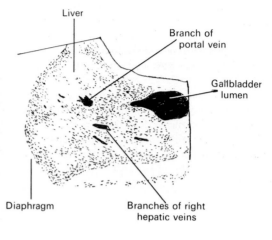

Liver

Branch of
portal vein

Gallbladder
lumen

Diaphragm

Branches of right
hepatic veins

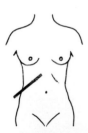

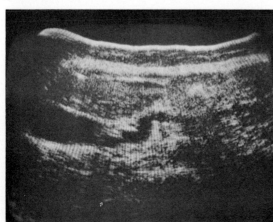

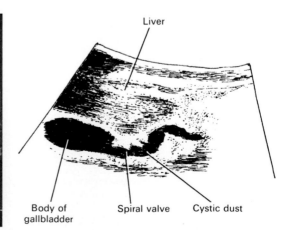

Liver

Body of
gallbladder

Spiral valve

Cystic dust

5.2 Gallbladder—normal anatomy

The gallbladder is most commonly an anterior relation to the right kidney and may be seen with the right kidney when scanned from the conventional posterior approach. This longitudinal ultrasonogram (upper figure) shows the right kidney with a physiologically distended gallbladder anterior to it.

Transverse sections through the gallbladder (lower figure) can be easily obtained through the intercostal spaces using the technique described on page 21 (Fig. 2.13). The transducer is placed in the intercostal space and small sector scans are carried out through the liver substance. This technique is extremely valuable in patients in whom there is gaseous distension of the colon and difficulty in visualizing the gallbladder from the anterior aspect. The liver may always be used as an acoustic window to demonstrate the gallbladder on transverse sections. The lower figure shows the gallbladder lumen lying anterior to the right kidney and embedded in the liver substance. The inferior vena cava and portal vein are seen more medially and the renal vessels may be seen draining into the inferior vena cava.

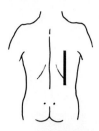

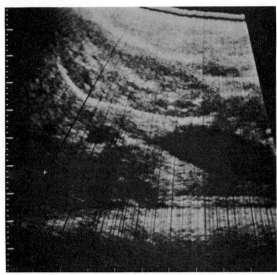

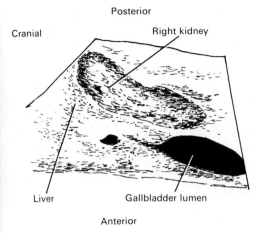

Posterior

Cranial   Right kidney

Liver   Gallbladder lumen

Anterior

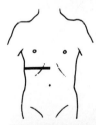

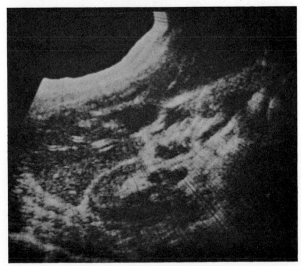

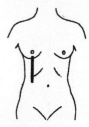

5.3 Gallstones

A 40-year-old female presented with transient attacks of right upper abdominal pain and intermittent jaundice. The biliary system failed to opacify on oral cholecystography.

A longitudinal ultrasonogram through the right lobe of the liver and gallbladder reveals the gallbladder lumen, which is of normal size. Multiple highly reflective opacities are seen within the gallbladder lumen, and these produce shadowing distal to them due to their high attenuation. These masses moved freely with gravity. Such appearances are characteristic of gallstones, and the diagnosis may be made with a high degree of confidence.

When all of these criteria are not met the diagnosis must be made with caution. Nonshadowing gallstones do occur, as shown in Figure 5.7; and the gallbladder lumen may not be visualized or be entirely filled with stones, as in Figure 5.8. An impacted gallstone may not move with gravity and may be confused with a papilloma or localized thickening of the gallbladder wall.

In summary, other appearances are consistent with the presence of gallstones, but the presence of reflective opacities within the lumen of the gallbladder which shadow distally and move with gravity are diagnostic of gallstones.

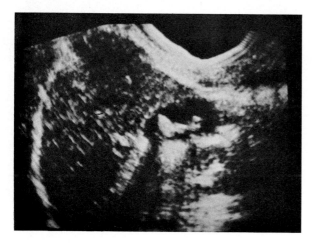

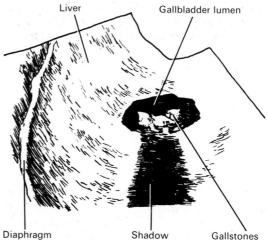

Liver   Gallbladder lumen

Diaphragm   Shadow   Gallstones

5.4 Congenital anomaly—septated gallbladder plus gallstones

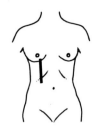

A septated gallbladder with contained gallstones was an incidental finding in a 65-year-old female referred for exclusion of metastatic disease to the liver. A definite line is seen passing through the lumen of the gallbladder. Two opacities are clearly seen in the gallbladder, and these produce distal shadowing due to high attenuation (absorption and scatter) within them. These masses also moved with gravity and show the classical appearances of gallstones.

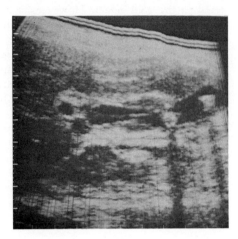
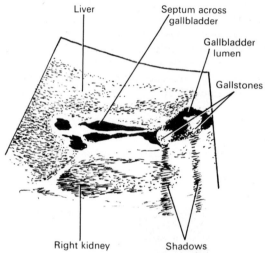

5.5 Gravel in the gallbladder

 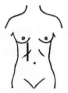 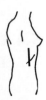

This 40-year-old female presented with symptoms of biliary tract disease. The ultrasound examination was carried out with the patient fasting.

A. Transverse ultrasonogram to show the gallbladder lumen which is physiologically dilated. The gallbladder is half full of fine particulate debris which shows no evidence of distal shadowing. Note that the pancreas and prevertebral vessels are well seen.

B. Paramedian ultrasonogram through the right upper quadrant to show the physiologically dilated gallbladder, which again, is half-full of particulate material. Note in both A and B the particulate matter layered under the influence of gravity. These patients should be examined in both the erect and left decubitus positions to determine whether the material contained within the gallbladder moves rapidly with gravity after changes in the patient's posture.

C. Ultrasonogram in the decubitus position. The particulate matter within the gallbladder has now layered in a new position, demonstrating that this is gravel and not sludge.

The significance of gravel in the gallbladder is still being evaluated. Sludge is certainly within the normal spectrum, but the presence of gravel suggests biliary tract disease and gallstones may be obscured by gravel. In a follow-up of 145 patients at this center, gallstones were found in only 60 percent of patients coming to surgery with non-shadowing material in the gallbladder. However, in the remaining 40 percent there was evidence of acute or chronic cholecystitis, either at surgery or on pathological examination. When these appearances are seen, one must also consider the possibility of empyema of the gallbladder, in which the particulate matter is due to pus within the gallbladder lumen. This must be excluded on clinical grounds.

Many patients with particulate matter within the gallbladder do not come to surgery because of absence of clinical symptoms and signs, and this particulate matter may pass spontaneously without symptoms. For this reason, the full significance of gravel has yet to be determined.

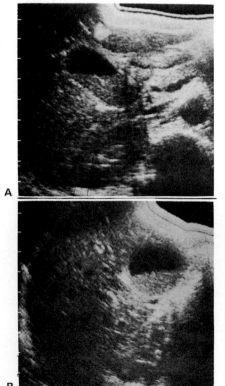

A

B

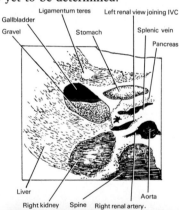

Ligamentum teres
Left renal view joining IVC
Gallbladder
Gravel
Stomach
Splenic vein
Pancreas
Liver
Aorta
Right kidney
Spine
Right renal artery

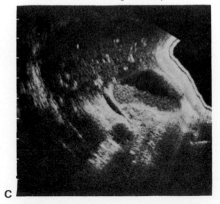

C

5.6 Gallbladder—sludge

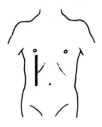

Sludge is not uncommon in the gallbladder, especially in alcoholics, and must be differentiated from gallstones. In this typical alcoholic patient, the gallbladder is large with a longitudinal axis of 12 cm, the extreme limit of normal. The dependent aspect of the gallbladder shows contained material which is fine in consistency but does not cause distal shadowing. When the patient was moved, the contained debris did not move with gravity, unlike gallstones and gravel. Sludge takes 20 to 30 minutes to move with gravity.

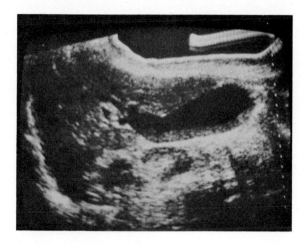
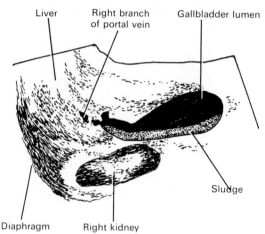

Liver   Right branch of portal vein   Gallbladder lumen

Diaphragm   Right kidney   Sludge

5.7 Nonshadowing gallstones plus debris

A. This 65-year-old male presented with a history highly suggestive of gallstones. On ultrasound examination with the patient fasting, a transverse section showed physiological dilatation of the gallbladder with opacities within the lumen but no marked distal shadowing. These opacities moved with gravity and appeared to be consistent with, but not classical of, the appearances of gallstones. At surgery, the gallbladder was found to contain multiple pigment stones.

B. This oblique ultrasonogram through the gallbladder lumen shows definite debris, which moved rapidly with gravity—thereby differentiating it from sludge. The material is, however, extremely fine and there is no evidence of shadowing distal to it. Similar appearances are seen with debris due to an empyema of the gallbladder (Fig. 5.9) or due to inspissated bile.

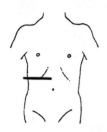

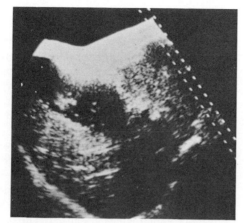

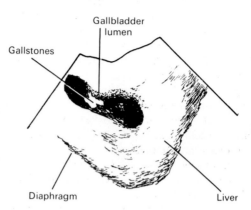

Gallbladder
lumen

Gallstones

Diaphragm

Liver

A

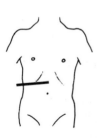

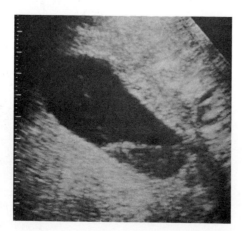

B

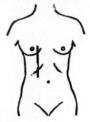

5.8 Small contracted gallbladder full of gallstones

Ultrasonic nonvisualization of the gallbladder lumen has been recently described—its pathological significance is still being assessed. In the fasting patient, physiological dilatation of the gallbladder should be observed, and if the gallbladder lumen is not demonstrated, three possibilities exist:

1. The gallbladder is congenitally absent. This has an incidence of only 0.03 percent.

2. The patient is not fasting and has eaten a fatty meal. This possibility can be checked by rescanning the patient after confirmed fasting.

3. The gallbladder is small and contracted, with a thickened wall, due to cholecystitis and is incapable of physiological distention.

Thus, in clinical practice, by far the commonest cause of ultrasonic nonvisualization of the gallbladder is the presence of a small and pathologically contracted gallbladder. Such gallbladders frequently contain stones and instead of the lumen being demonstrated, a highly reflective opacity is seen within the gallbladder fossa, and there is distal shadowing. In our series to date, of 25 patients coming to surgery, 24 were found to have chronic inflammatory changes producing a shrunken gallbladder with gallstones.

A. This 40-year-old female presented with symptoms suggesting biliary tract disease. There was nonvisualization of the gallbladder on oral cholecystography.

This paramedian section 6 cm to the right of the midline shows a reflective opacity apparently within the liver substance, which shadows markedly across the upper pole of the right kidney. No evidence was found of physiological dilatation of the gallbladder. The changes of chronic cholecystitis and gallstones were found at surgery.

B. This transverse ultrasonogram shows the appearances of nonvisualization of the gallbladder on ultrasound examination. A reflective and shadowing opacity is seen anterior to the right kidney, just lateral to the head of the pancreas. The normal gallbladder lumen is not visualized. The pancreas and great vessels are well demonstrated.

In such patients it is important to differentiate between air in the duodenum causing a shadow, and pathology of the gallbladder producing a shadow. Again, it is the absence of the normal gallbladder lumen which indicates definite pathology.

C. This is a further example of ultrasonic nonvisualization of the gallbladder lumen. An opacity is seen in the gallbladder fossa which shadows distally.

D. Surgical specimen of small, contracted gallbladder and gallstones from the patient scanned in Figure C.

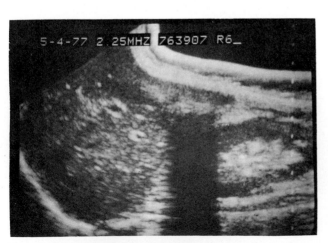

5-4-77 2.25MHZ 763907 R6_

A

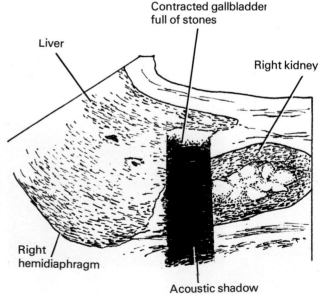

Contracted gallbladder full of stones

Liver

Right kidney

Right hemidiaphragm

Acoustic shadow

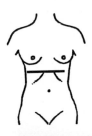

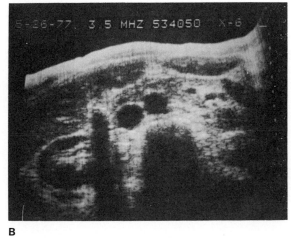

B

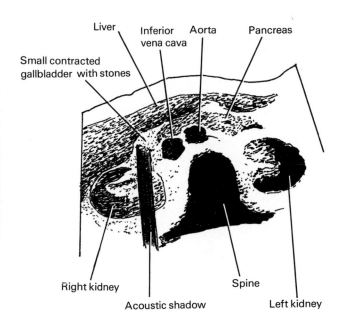

Small contracted
gallbladder with stones

Liver   Inferior   Aorta   Pancreas
        vena cava

Right kidney   Spine   Left kidney

Acoustic shadow

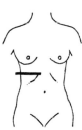

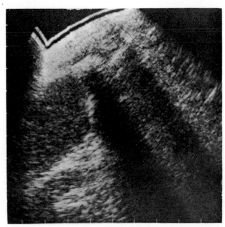

C

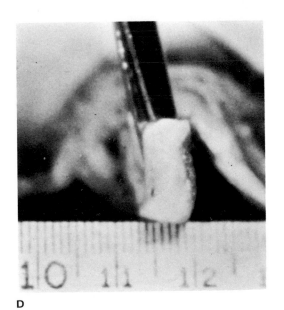

D

5.9 Empyema of the gallbladder

This 44-year-old female presented with an unknown septic focus. Transverse ultrasound examination through the gallbladder fossa (upper figure) using an intercostal sector scan shows the gallbladder lumen half full of fine cellular debris. Such appearances may be due to an empyema of the gallbladder, but any other fine and granular contents of the gallbladder may simulate these appearances.

A further transverse section through the gallbladder (lower figure) shows the gallbladder with a further fluid-filled cavity within the liver substance, and this raises the possibility of an abscess cavity surrounding the gallbladder—suggesting that this is an empyema of the gallbladder with spread to the surrounding tissues.

At surgery, an empyema of the gallbladder was removed and the gallbladder lumen was noted to be ruptured.

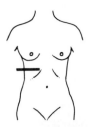

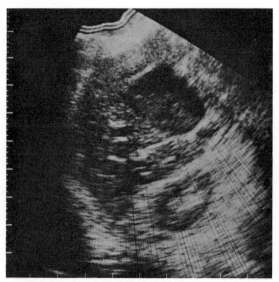

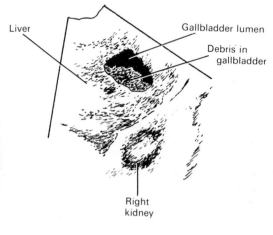

Liver

Gallbladder lumen

Debris in gallbladder

Right kidney

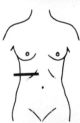

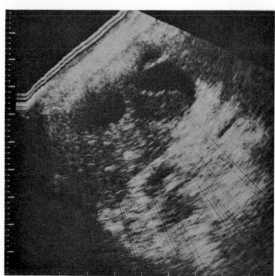

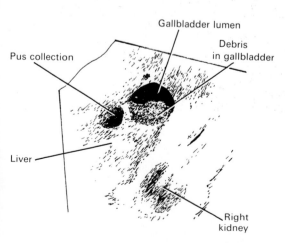

Gallbladder lumen

Debris in gallbladder

Pus collection

Liver

Right kidney

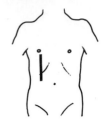

5.10 Hydrops of gallbladder

A. A 43-year-old male was known to suffer from Hodgkin's disease and presented with a mobile, palpable mass in the right hypochondrium. The ultrasonogram, taken in the paramedian plane 6 cm to the right of the midline, shows the palpable mass to be pyriform in shape and cystic in nature. There is a definite shadow thrown from the neck of the gallbladder, which is found in all gallbladders and is not due to a gallstone impacted in the neck. The gallbladder does appear to be obstructed from its shape and state of distention. The appearances are consistent with those of a mucocele of the gallbladder.

B. This paramedian ultrasonogram shows marked dilatation of the gallbladder, the longitudinal axis measuring 16 cm. In the author's experience to date, 12 cm is the upper limit of normal. However, many hydrops of the gallbladder will be smaller than this.

C. Transverse ultrasonogram of the same patient as that shown in Figure 5.10B. A markedly distended gallbladder is seen lying anterior to the right kidney. Note the very constant relationship between the gallbladder lumen, the duodenum which contains an air bubble, and the head of the pancreas passing from the lateral to the medial aspect.

At surgery, hydrops of the gallbladder due to a stone impacted in the cystic duct, was confirmed. Such stones are usually missed on ultrasound examination.

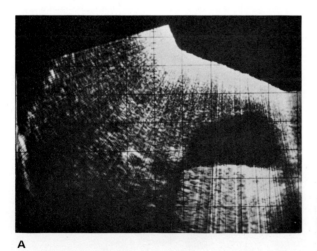

A

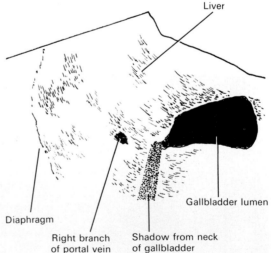

Liver

Gallbladder lumen

Diaphragm

Right branch
of portal vein

Shadow from neck
of gallbladder

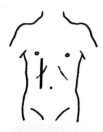

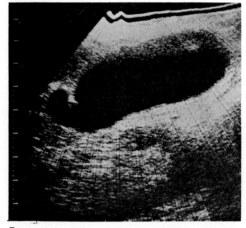

B

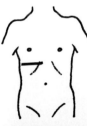

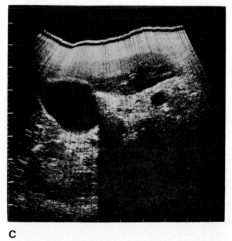

C

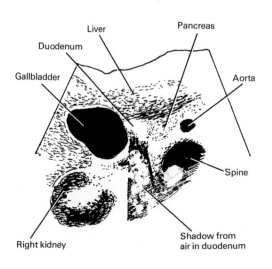

Liver

Duodenum

Pancreas

Gallbladder

Aorta

Spine

Right kidney

Shadow from
air in duodenum

5.11 Acute hydrops of gallbladder in a child

A 4-year-old child was admitted with a history of fever of seven days' duration of 40°C (104°F) and treated successfully with oral and intramuscular penicillin. On admission, cervical lymphadenopathy and an erythematous throat were noted, but there was no abnormality in the abdomen. During the course of the next three days, a palpable mass became apparent in the right hypochondrium and this appeared to be a tense, distended gallbladder. The ultrasound examination shows a distended gallbladder on longitudinal section (upper figure) and transverse section (lower figure). At surgery the ultrasound findings of hydrops of the gallbladder were confirmed and the patient treated by cholecystostomy and cholecystectomy.

No gallstones were present and obstruction of the cystic duct was due to inspissation of bile associated with prolonged pyrexia and dehydration. Physiological distension must be differentiated from hydrops. A tense gallbladder which can be ballotted on palpation is evidence of pathological tension. If doubts exists, the patient should be reexamined after a fatty meal.

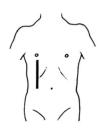

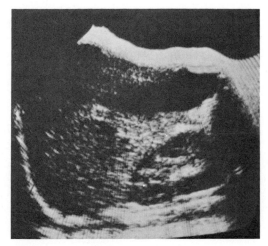

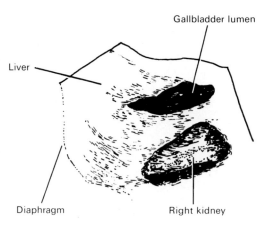

Gallbladder lumen

Liver

Diaphragm

Right kidney

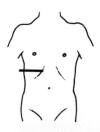

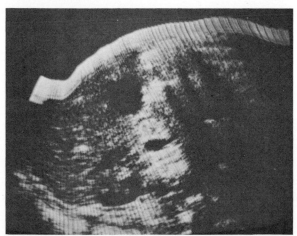

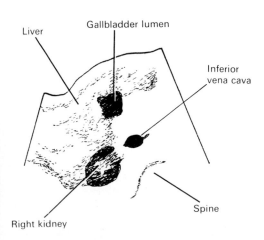

Liver

Gallbladder lumen

Inferior vena cava

Right kidney

Spine

5.12 Distended cystic duct and gallbladder

This elderly male was referred for ultrasonic examination of the biliary tree following episodes of fever and right upper quadrant pain which simulated acute cholecystitis. An oblique subcostal scan (upper figure) in the plane of the subcostal margin shows the gallbladder fundus and body along its longitudinal axis, converging into the neck of the gallbladder and passing into a dilated cystic duct. This duct is 1.5 cm in diameter and the mucosal folds can be seen in the wall of the duct, which forms part of the spiral valve. This spiral valve is optimally seen in a slightly lower section through the gallbladder lumen (lower figure).

Surgery revealed an obstructed cystic duct due to a cholangiocarcinoma.

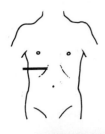

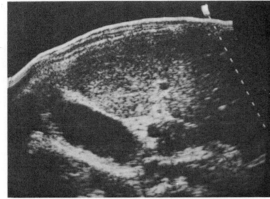

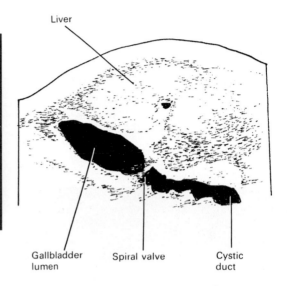

Liver

Gallbladder
lumen

Spiral valve

Cystic
duct

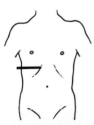

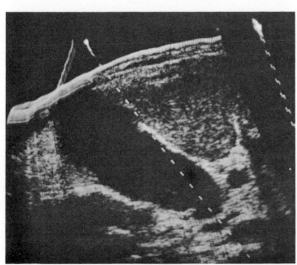

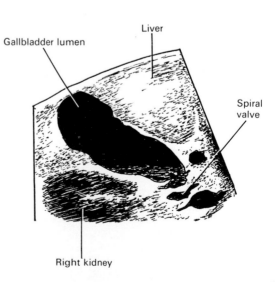

Gallbladder lumen

Liver

Spiral
valve

Right kidney

117

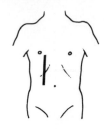

5.13 Gallbladder—spherical shape in extrahepatic biliary obstruction

This 65-year-old male presented with obstructive jaundice due to a carcinoma of the head of the pancreas. Dilated intrahepatic biliary canaliculi are seen throughout the liver substance in the parasagittal ultrasonogram. The gallbladder is only 4 cm in length but is abnormally spherical in contour, suggesting obstruction and abnormal tension. Due to the wide variation in the size of the gallbladder, the shape of the gallbladder or the state of the intrahepatic canalculi are of greater importance in diagnosing biliary obstruction. If there is cause for doubt as to whether a gallbladder shows physiological distention or there is an obstructed hydrops of the gallbladder, the patient can be rescanned after milk or a fatty meal.

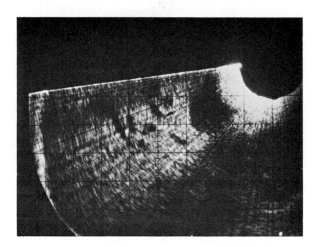

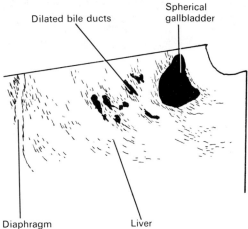

Dilated bile ducts

Spherical gallbladder

Diaphragm

Liver

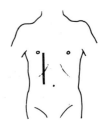

5.14 Extrahepatic biliary obstruction

A 45-year-old male had been treated with surgery and radiotherapy for a primary seminoma. On follow-up, he complained of the recent onset of jaundice which was found to be cholestatic in type. The main differential lay between metastatic disease of the liver and obstruction to the extrahepatic biliary tree by involved para-aortic nodes. An ultrasonogram was performed and this paramedian section taken 6 cm to the right of the midline shows a moderately distended gallbladder, but there is very definite dilatation of the intrahepatic biliary vessels. These dilated vessels could be traced as far as the porta hepatis, clearly inferring that there was an extrahepatic cause for the obstruction below the porta hepatis. The precise cause could not be visualized due to air in the gut and fibrosis from previous radiotherapy. On these results, surgery was indicated. At surgery, involved lymph nodes were found of mixed histology in the upper para-aortic position, and there was distention of the biliary tree which was relieved by a choledochojejunostomy. The gallbladder did not communicate with the biliary tree, accounting for its modest size. A metastasis is apparent above the gallbladder.

The gallbladder size is not an adequate indicator of biliary obstruction since it may be relatively normal, as in this case, or it may be grossly dilated, forming a mucocele without obstruction to the whole biliary tree.

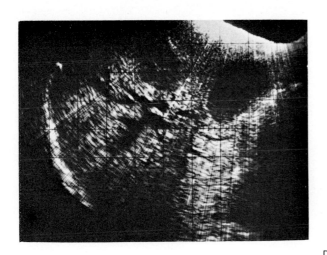

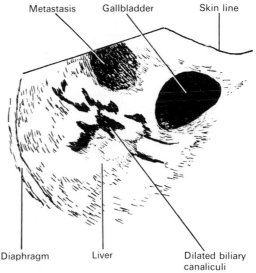

Metastasis   Gallbladder   Skin line

Diaphragm   Liver   Dilated biliary canaliculi

5.15 Extrahepatic biliary obstruction due to lymphadenopathy

A 56-year-old male suffered from immunoblastic lymphadenopathy and developed jaundice which was cholestatic in type. A paramedian ultrasonogram (upper figure) taken 6 cm to the right of the midline shows a distended gallbladder in addition to dilated biliary canaliculi throughout the liver substance. The cause for this was found in a more medial section through the region of the porta hepatis in a paramedian section taken 3 cm to the right of the midline (lower figure). This shows a lobulated mass which appears to invaginate itself into the liver substance; these appearances are compatible with lymphadenopathy at the porta hepatis. This may occasionally cause obstruction to the extrahepatic biliary tree.

The gallbladder is highly variable in size and may occasionally be up to 12 cm in length. Therefore, the shape of the gallbladder is of more importance in attempting to diagnose obstruction. Note that the gallbladder is more spherical than usual, suggesting tension. The patient may be rescanned after a fatty meal to give further evidence of biliary obstruction.

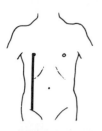

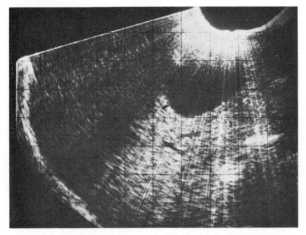

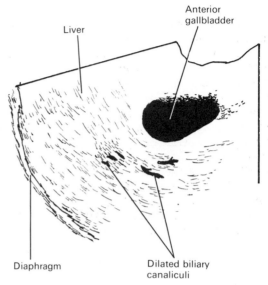

Liver

Anterior
gallbladder

Diaphragm

Dilated biliary
canaliculi

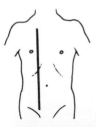

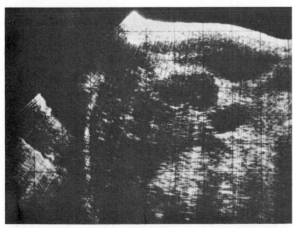

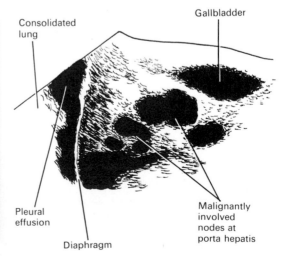

Consolidated
lung

Gallbladder

Pleural
effusion

Diaphragm

Malignantly
involved
nodes at
porta hepatis

121

5.16 Metabolic—extrahepatic biliary obstruction due to gallstones

This 55-year-old female presented with cholestatic jaundice and was referred for ultrasound to determine whether this was intra- or extrahepatic in site. A parasagittal ultrasonogram through the right lobe of the liver (upper figure) shows a normal liver substance except for dilated biliary canaliculi. The gallbladder is easily indentified and contains at least one large gallstone, which appears as a highly reflective opacity in the gallbladder lumen and casts a shadow distal to it.

A more medial scan, 2 cm to the left of the midline (lower figure), shows the inferior vena cava posteriorly with a large dilated tube more anteriorly. Note that just below the porta hepatis this tube shows a small anterior deviation but is otherwise straight and parallel with the inferior vena cava. These are the characteristics of the common bile duct. Compared with the common bile duct, an enlarged portal vein is tortuous and penetrates more deeply into the liver (p. 77).

The dilated common bile duct can be traced almost to its termination in the duodenum, but the precise cause of the obstruction cannot be seen. At surgery an impacted stone was found. Small stones are seen in the upper part of the dilated duct. Gallstones can, of course, coincide with other causes of biliary obstruction, including tumors and structures.

Anterior to the inferior vena cava is a very reliable site to search for dilatation of the intrahepatic biliary vessels. The configuration seen here is not mimicked by dilatation of the blood vessels.

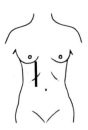

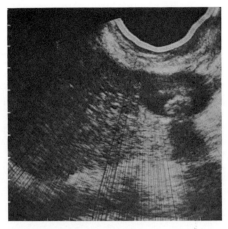

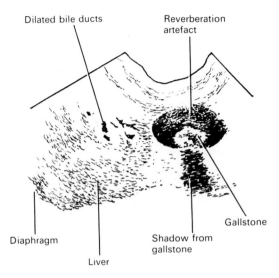

Dilated bile ducts

Reverberation artefact

Diaphragm

Liver

Shadow from gallstone

Gallstone

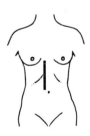

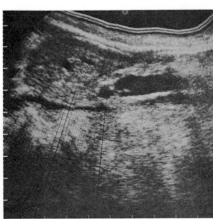

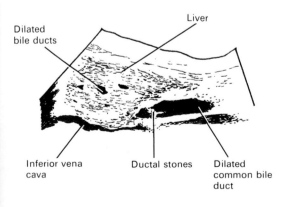

Liver

Dilated bile ducts

Inferior vena cava

Ductal stones

Dilated common bile duct

5.17 Gallstones in the common bile duct

This 54-year-old female presented with right upper quadrant pain and sudden onset of jaundice, obstructive in nature. The paramedian ultrasound section 2 cm to the right of the midline (upper figure) shows a dilated tube, the common bile duct lying anterior and parallel to the inferior vena cava. A definite opacity is seen within the duct which casts a shadow distal to the opacity. These appearances indicate the presence of a ductal stone. Dilatation of the whole of the common bile duct implies a further obstruction at the ampulla. The liver substance shows distention of the intrahepatic biliary canaliculi.

A transverse section (lower figure) shows the lumen of the gallbladder immediately lateral to the dilated common bile duct. Both contain stones. At surgery, gallstones were found in the gallbladder and common bile duct, and impacted in the ampulla.

In the experience of the author, intravenous cholangiography is the method of choice to display common duct stones. The tomographic nature of the imaging process both by ultrasound and by CT make it easy to miss small stones.

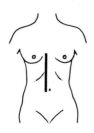

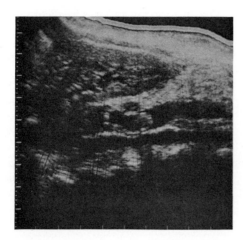

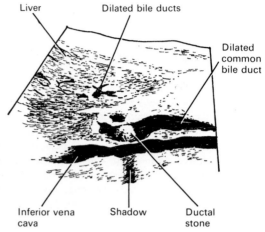

Liver   Dilated bile ducts

Dilated common bile duct

Inferior vena cava   Shadow   Ductal stone

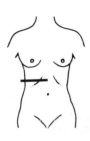

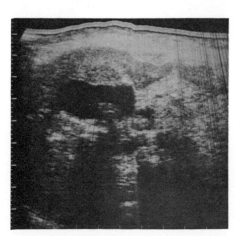

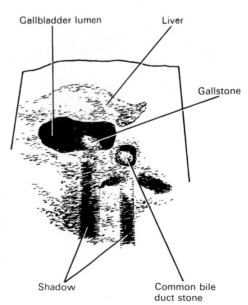

Gallbladder lumen   Liver

Gallstone

Shadow   Common bile duct stone

5.18 Extrahepatic obstruction to common bile duct

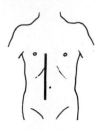

A 55-year-old man presented with a history of upper abdominal pain and the recent onset of jaundice which was cholestatic in type. The ultrasound scan in the region of the porta hepatis is shown in the longitudinal scan. A dilated tube can be seen lying immediately anterior to the inferior vena cava. The configuration of this implies that this can only be the common bile duct which can be traced to its drainage into the duodenum. Thus the cause of the jaundice was extrahepatic due to an obstruction at the ampulla of Vater. The apparent shadow at the lower end of the common bile duct suggested that this was due to a stone impacted at the ampulla, but surgery revealed that the stone was impacted at that site due to a stenosis resulting from a carcinoma of the ampulla.

Due to air in the gut, it is frequently not possible to display the common bile duct, even when it is dilated, so that the diagnosis of an extrahepatic cause for biliary obstruction must rest on observations on the state of the intrahepatic biliary vessels. There are definite dilated vessels within the liver substance, and the H shape seen in the region of the porta hepatis is characteristic of an extrahepatic cause for obstruction. Once an extrahepatic cause has been demonstrated, surgery is virtually always indicated, and the important contribution which can be made by the ultrasonologist is the highly accurate differentiation between intra- and extrahepatic causes for biliary obstruction. At this center, an accuracy of 96 % has been achieved in this application.

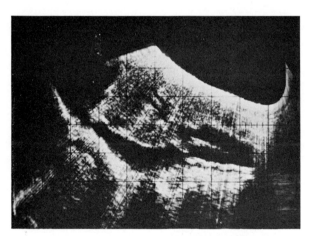

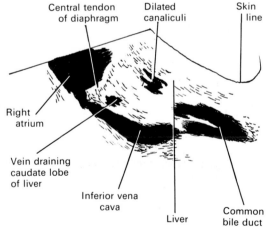

Central tendon of diaphragm — Dilated canaliculi — Skin line — Right atrium — Vein draining caudate lobe of liver — Inferior vena cava — Liver — Common bile duct

5.19 Extrahepatic obstruction due to carcinoma of the pancreas

A 60-year-old male presented with painless jaundice of three weeks' duration. Transverse (A) and longitudinal (B) sections through the liver reveal marked distention of the intrahepatic biliary canaliculi, indicating an extrahepatic site of biliary obstruction.

A longitudinal section 2 cm to the right of the midline (B) shows a dilated common bile duct containing small stones, and this duct can be traced inferiorly for 7 cm before ending in an ill-defined mass partially obscured by intestinal gas. The common bile duct and entire biliary tree is therefore obstructed in the region of the pancreas. A transhepatic cholangiogram was unsuccessful, but laparotomy revealed a small carcinoma of the head of the pancreas causing biliary obstruction.

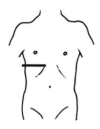

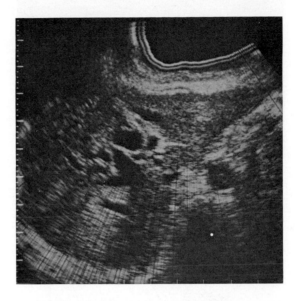

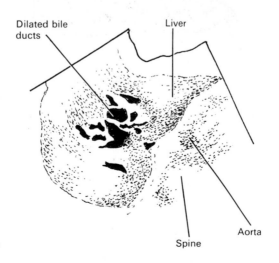

Dilated bile ducts

Liver

Spine

Aorta

A

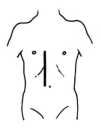

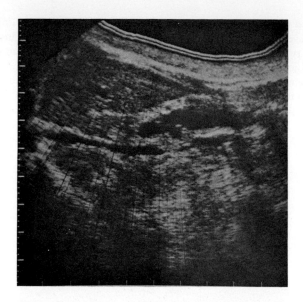

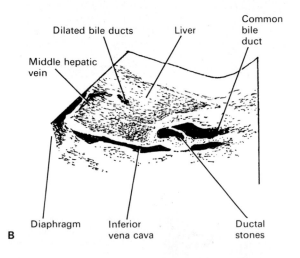

Dilated bile ducts   Liver   Common bile duct

Middle hepatic vein

Diaphragm   Inferior vena cava   Ductal stones

B

5.20 Jaundice due to lymphomatous infiltration of the liver

A 35-year-old male, known to suffer from a non-Hodgkin's lymphoma, became jaundiced. Biochemical examination showed this to be cholestatic in type. The differential diagnosis lay between malignant infiltration of the liver, other hepatic causes of jaundice, and obstruction to the larger ducts of the biliary system due to involved lymph nodes. A paramedian ultrasonogram (A) shows the inferior vena cava in length; the portal vein is a little large as frequently occurs when there is extensive liver involvement by tumor. However, there is no evidence of a dilated common bile duct. A more lateral section (B) taken 6 cm to the right of the midline confirms hepatomegaly, and small discrete tumor areas are seen throughout the liver substance. The right kidney is seen posteriorly. There is no evidence of dilated biliary vessels. These scans imply that cholestatic jaundice was due to malignant involvement of the liver, and there was no evidence of extrahepatic biliary obstruction.

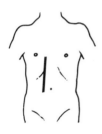

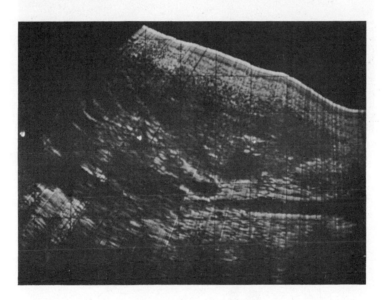

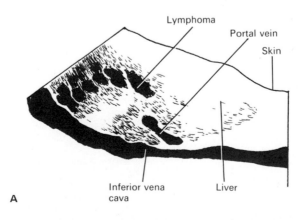

Lymphoma

Portal vein

Skin

Inferior vena cava

Liver

A

129

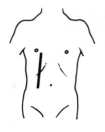
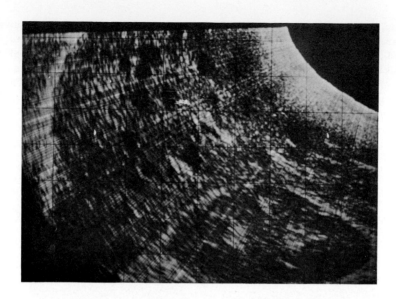
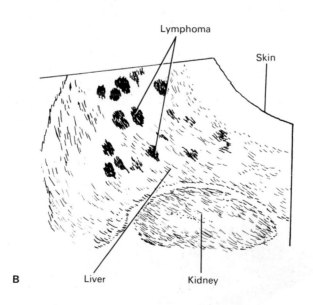

Lymphoma

Skin

Liver

Kidney

B

130

6. The pancreas °

6.1 Examination technique

Patients are examined as early as possible in the morning in a fasting state, thus minimizing the problem of intestinal gas and allowing effective examination of the gallbladder and biliary tract simultaneously. This simple preparation permits a successful exam in about 90% of patients. An intestinal purge may be helpful in the remaining patients, especially those in whom a suspicious mass is seen in the tail of the pancreas which might be confused with colon contents. Patients are examined in deep suspended inspiration so that the descent of the liver anterior to the pancreas displaces bowel gas and provides a good acoustic window to the prevertebral region. Deep inspiration also dilates the venous structures, which is important in localizing the pancreas.

Since the pancreas is transversely oriented and moves in a cephalocaudad direction with respiration, it is especially important to obtain sagittal sections so the organ is optimally demonstrated. Examination is begun with a right parasagittal section over the inferior vena cava, locating the head of the pancreas. It lies on the anterior surface of the IVC, just caudal to the crossing of the IVC by the portal vein. Next, the neck and body of the pancreas are located anterior to the mesenteric vessels in a parasagittal section of the aorta. The celiac trunk and its branches are used to define the cephalad limit of the pancreas. Noting the position of the pancreas from the sagittal scans, a proper oblique transverse scan is performed through the long axis of the pancreas usually visualizing its entire length. Since intestinal gas in the left upper quadrant often obscures visualization of the tail of the pancreas, it should be examined with the patient prone using the left kidney as an acoustic window.

In the average patient a 2.25 megahertz transducer focused at 7–9 cm is used. When possible in thin patients a 3.5 megahertz 13 mm transducer focused at 5–7 cm will provide better resolution.

6.2 Normal anatomy

The pancreas is a transversely oriented retroperitoneal organ which is intimately related to the upper abdominal vasculature. Recent improvements in the gray scale technique allow the identification of the vascular anatomy and greatly improve the demonstration of the pancreas by ultrasonic techniques. Although echoes from normal pancreatic tissue are demonstrated only in about 70 % of patients, with knowledge of the vascular anatomy, one can conclude that the pancreas is of normal size by knowing that the space it occupies is not enlarged.

The relationship of the pancreas to the vascular anatomy is represented diagramatically in Figure 6.2A in transverse section. Anatomically, the pancreas is divided into the head, neck, body and tail. The head of the pancreas is bordered laterally by the second portion of the duodenum and lies just anterior to the inferior vena cava. The pancreas extends ventral to the aorta and superior mesenteric vessels, the latter forming a groove in the posterior surface of the pancreas marking the anatomic neck. At this point, the splenic vein, which normally courses in a groove on the posterior surface of the pancreas, can be seen joining the superior mesenteric vein to form the portal vein. The body of the pancreas courses to the left of the spine and posteriorly to rest just anterior to the left kidney and continues as the tail, ending near the hilum of the spleen. The left renal vein can be seen coursing between the superior mesenteric artery and the aorta to join the inferior vena cava, providing another vascular landmark in transverse section.

Figures 6.2B and C demonstrates the anatomic correlation by angiography. In Figure B a selective celiac injection demonstrates contrast flow through the pancreaticoduodenal arcades, outlining the head of the pancreas, with flash filling of the origin of the superior mesenteric artery. The pancreatic outline is superimposed on the spine and the origin of the superior mesenteric artery. Note that its cephalad limit is the celiac trunk and its branches the hepatic and splenic arteries. Figure 6.2C, the venous phase of the same angiogram, shows the course of the splenic vein which runs posterior to the body of the pancreas to form the portal vein behind the neck. This junction can be correlated with the arteriographic phase in Figure 6.2B. Note that the head of the pancreas, which is well outlined on the arteriographic phase, is located just caudal to the portal vein. Thus, a sagittal section along the inferior vena cava will locate the head of the pancreas just caudal to the crossing of the portal vein and the inferior vena cava.

This angiographic anatomy is correlated with the ultrasound sagittal sections in Figures 6.2D and E. In Figure 6.2D the head of the pancreas is located just caudal to the portal vein and in Figure 6.2E the body of the pancreas is located between the superior mesenteric vein and the left lobe of the liver, with its cephalad limit being defined by the splenic artery. The transverse section in Figure 6.2F (arrowed) shows the pancreas anterior to the superior mesenteric vein and artery and the left renal vein coursing between the aorta and the SMA. In Figure 6.2G the typical appearance of the tail of the pancreas is seen in a sagittal section through the left kidney with the patient in the prone position.

More detailed anatomy can occasionally be seen and Figure 6.2H shows two sagittal sections over the aorta (upper) and the inferior vena cava (lower). In the upper section the superior mesenteric vein, with its bulbous cephalad termination, is well visualized with pancreatic tissue located between it and the left lobe of the liver. The splenic artery and left renal vein are seen in cross section. The section below demonstrates more detailed anatomy of the head of the pancreas. The gastroduodenal artery courses along the anterior surface of the head of the pancreas, whereas the common duct is on the posterior surface. This same anatomy is seen in Figure 6.2J which represents a detailed transverse section of the head of the pancreas. Note the superior mesenteric vein, left renal vein entering the vena cava, and within the head of the pancreas two small round structures which represent the gastroduodenal artery (upper) and the common duct (lower). An enlarged transverse cross section is seen in Figure 6.2K and demonstrates the diffuse fine echo pattern of the normal pancreas. The pancreas should be at least as echogenic or more echogenic than the liver and variation from this normal consistency indicates pathology. The size of the normal pancreas has been variously reported in the literature and has been measured in different ways. If repeatable examinations are to be made using easily located vascular landmarks, sagittal sections should be employed to measure the largest AP diameter. Presently it is felt that 2 cm is the upper limit of normal for the head of the pancreas, representing the thickest portion.

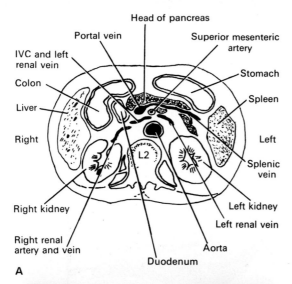

Head of pancreas

Portal vein

Superior mesenteric artery

IVC and left renal vein

Stomach

Colon

Spleen

Liver

Right

Left

Splenic vein

L2

Right kidney

Left kidney

Left renal vein

Right renal artery and vein

Aorta

Duodenum

A

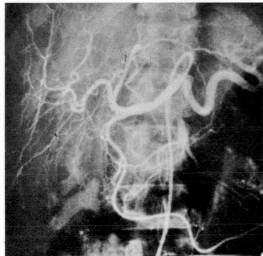

B

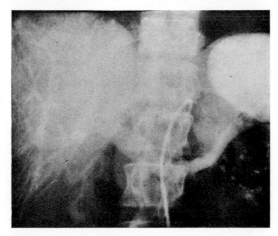

C

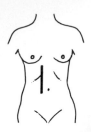

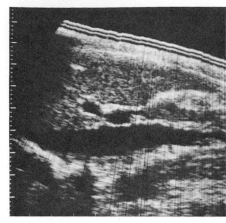

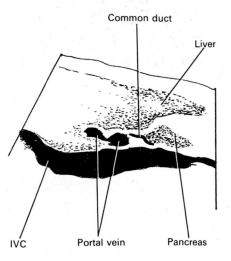

D

Common duct

Liver

IVC

Portal vein

Pancreas

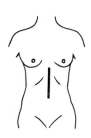

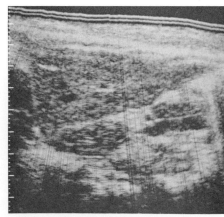

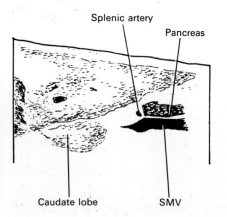

E

Splenic artery

Pancreas

Caudate lobe

SMV

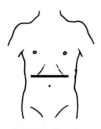

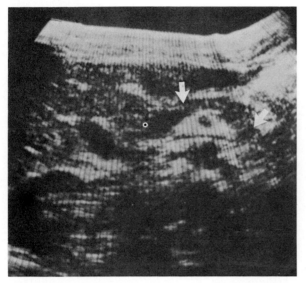

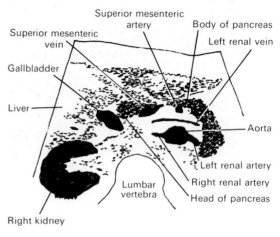

Superior mesenteric
artery

Superior mesenteric
vein

Body of pancreas

Left renal vein

Gallbladder

Liver

Aorta

Left renal artery

Right renal artery

Head of pancreas

Lumbar
vertebra

Right kidney

F

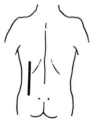

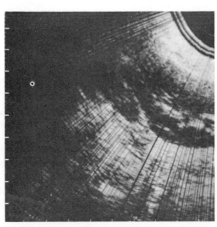

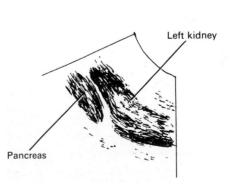

Left kidney

Pancreas

G

135

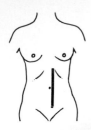

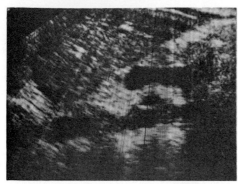

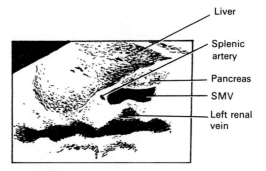

Liver
Splenic artery
Pancreas
SMV
Left renal vein

H (upper)

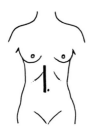

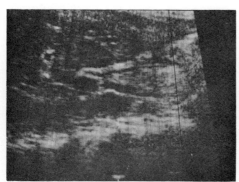

Liver
Gastroduodenal artery
Pancreas
Common duct

H (lower)

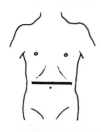

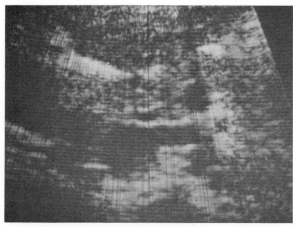

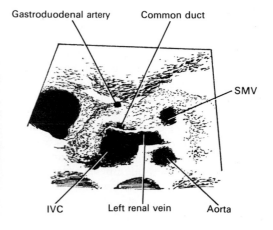

Gastroduodenal artery   Common duct

SMV

IVC   Left renal vein   Aorta

J

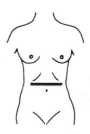

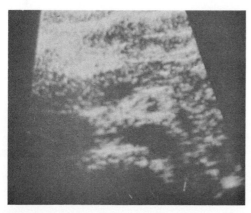

K

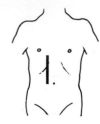

6.3 Acute pancreatitis

This middle-aged alcoholic with acute pancreatitis demonstrates diffuse enlargement of the head, neck, body and tail of the pancreas. Note that in addition to the enlargement of the organ, it returns lower level internal echoes than the liver, indicating edema of the pancreas. The diagnosis of pancreatitis is made both on the criterion of a diffuse enlargement of the gland as well as on a decrease in echogenicity. When there is only a localized enlargement of the gland, the differentiation between localized pancreatitis and carcinoma may be difficult. Then, observing the more prominent attenuation of carcinoma may allow this differentiation.

In Figure 6.3A, a parasagittal section over the inferior vena cava shows the marked compression of its anterior surface by an enlarged head of the pancreas, which measures about 4 cm. Figure 6.3B represents a sagittal section over the aorta demonstrating the body of the pancreas lying between the left lobe of the liver and the superior mesenteric vein. Figure 6.3C again demonstrates the superior mesenteric artery and superior mesenteric vein with the pancreas lying just anterior to them. Vascular structures seen on end just cephalad to the superior mesenteric artery represent branches of the celiac trunk, marking the most cephalad limit of the pancreas. Transverse scans (Figs. 6.3D and E) demonstrate a diffuse enlargement of the gland. The left renal vein is seen passing between the superior mesenteric artery and the aorta and the vena cava is seen as a slit-like structure due to the compression from the enlarged pancreas.

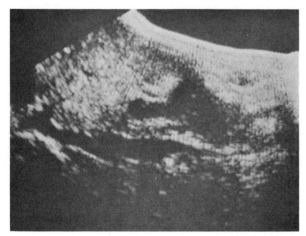

A

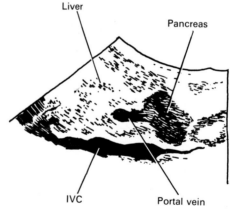

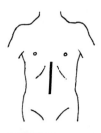

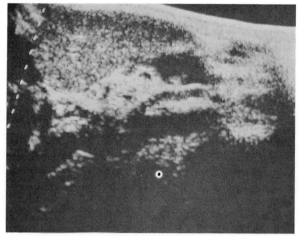

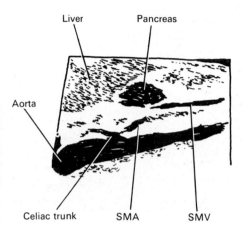

Liver   Pancreas

Aorta

Celiac trunk   SMA   SMV

B

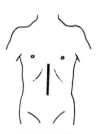

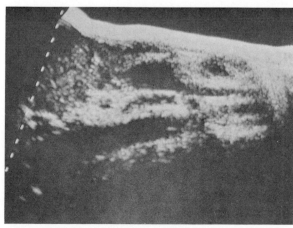

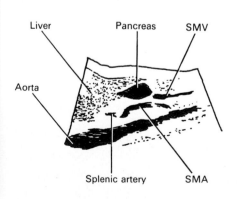

Liver   Pancreas   SMV

Aorta

Splenic artery   SMA

C

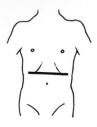

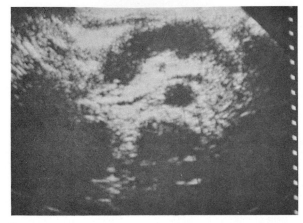

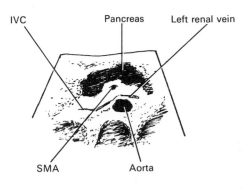

D

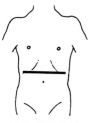

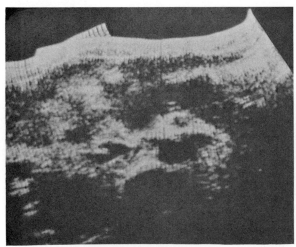

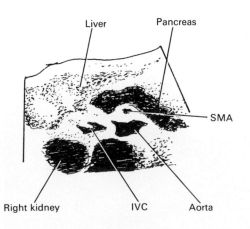

E

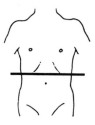

6.4 Acute on chronic pancreatitis

This transverse ultrasonogram shows diffuse enlargement of the head and body of the pancreas which also has an abnormal consistency. Most of the gland returns lower level echoes than the liver substance and this is consistent with edema in acute pancreatitis. In addition, there are areas of high-level echoes appearing as white flecks, especially in the head. This suggests fibrosis in the gland and these appearances are characteristic of acute pancreatitis superimposed on chronic inflammatory disease.

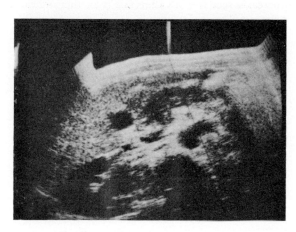

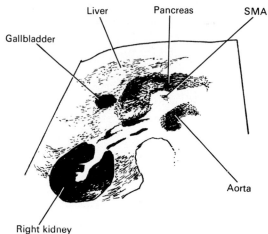

6.5 Chronic pancreatitis

This 40-year-old chronic alcoholic with a long history of recurrent pancreatitis entered the hospital with a mild acute exacerbation. A transverse echogram (upper) demonstrates a diffusely enlarged gland but with relatively stronger internal echoes than normal, indicative of chronic inflammatory change, probably secondary to fibrosis in the gland. Again note the superior mesenteric artery and vein which are landmarks for the pancreas. A sagittal section (lower) of the aorta demonstrates the vertically oriented celiac trunk and the origin of the superior mesenteric artery just caudad. The pancreas lies between the superior mesenteric artery and the left lobe of the liver and immediately anterior to the splenic vein, which is seen in cross section. Note that the celiac trunk marks the cephalad limit of the pancreas. The irregular margin of the pancreas is seen in both scans and is another indication of chronic change.

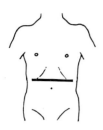

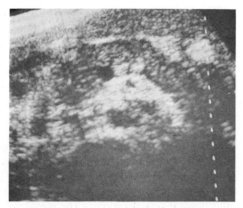

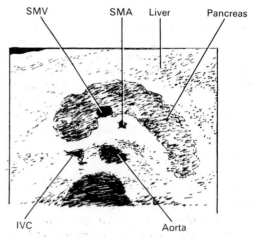

SMV   SMA   Liver   Pancreas

IVC   Aorta

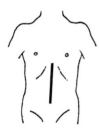

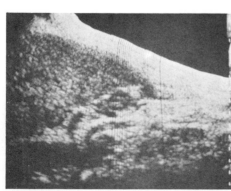

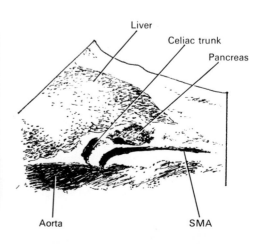

Liver

Celiac trunk

Pancreas

Aorta   SMA

143

6.6 Localized mass in chronic pancreatitis

This 40-year-old chronic male alcoholic presented with painless jaundice and weight loss. A sagittal echogram (Fig. 6.6A) above the inferior vena cava reveals marked compression by a large mass within the head of the pancreas returning echoes of the same amplitude as the liver. A second sagittal section (Fig. 6.6B) above the mesenteric vessels also demonstrates marked enlargement of the neck and body of the pancreas. A transverse echogram (Fig. 6.6C) shows an ill-defined, relatively localized mass in the head and body of the pancreas. In Figure 6.6D there is dilatation of the intrahepatic biliary tree and a normal-sized gallbladder without evidence of calculi. However, the rounded shape of the gallbladder suggests that it is obstructed. An oblique sagittal scan (Fig. 6.6E) demonstrates the dilated common duct down to the level of the mass in the head of the pancreas. Note that the dilated common duct passes anterior to the portal vein. Normally the common duct descends more posteriorly behind the head of the pancreas, but because of the large mass its distal part is elevated anteriorly in this patient. A second oblique sagittal scan (Fig. 6.6F) along the axis of the portal vein is shown for comparison, demonstrating its typical course ending in an upward

"C" configuration as it enters the hilum of the liver.

Because of a strong suspicion of carcinoma, an endoscopic retrograde cholangio-pancreatography (ERCP) (Fig. 6.6G) was performed demonstrating the classic changes of pancreatitis with a long stricture in the assessory duct which traversed the region of the mass. A transhepatic cholangiogram (Fig. 6.6H) also revealed a long, benign-appearing stricture of the distal common duct.

A cross table lateral view of the transhepatic cholangiogram (Fig. 6.6J) provides a correlation with the ultrasound scan of the common duct. Figure 6.6K shows the venous phase of a superior mesenteric artery injection for opacification of the portal vein. Note the correlation with the ultrasound scan of the portal vein (Fig. 6.6F). Thus the course of the common duct and portal vein differ substantially and should not be confused.

At surgery the patient was found to have a large inflammatory mass without evidence of tumor. Drainage of the biliary tree and pancreatic duct were accomplished by anastomosis to the small bowel.

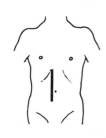

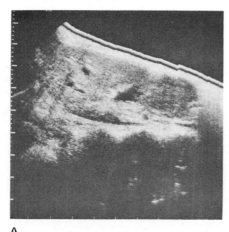

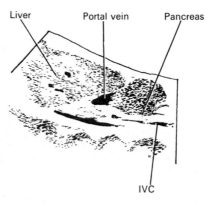

Liver   Portal vein   Pancreas

IVC

A

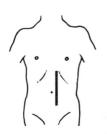

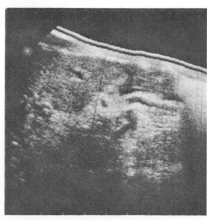

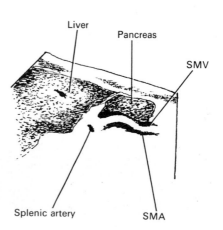

Liver   Pancreas

SMV

Splenic artery   SMA

B

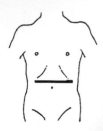

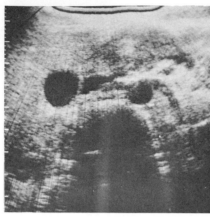

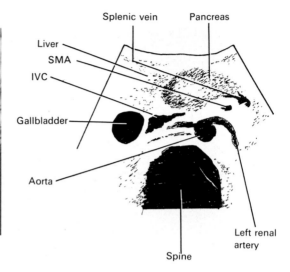

Splenic vein   Pancreas

Liver

SMA

IVC

Gallbladder

Aorta

Spine

Left renal artery

C

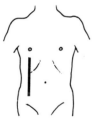

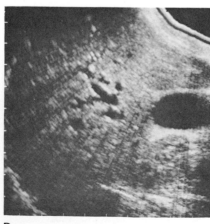

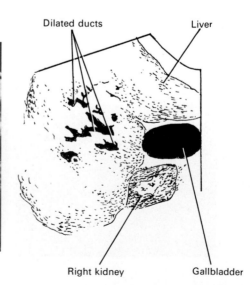

Dilated ducts   Liver

Right kidney   Gallbladder

D

146

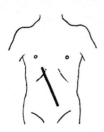

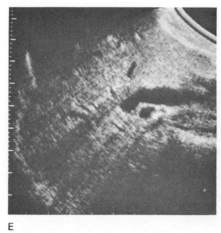

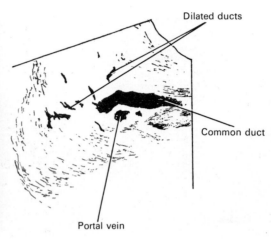

Dilated ducts

Common duct

Portal vein

E

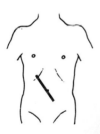

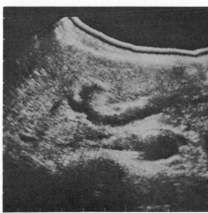

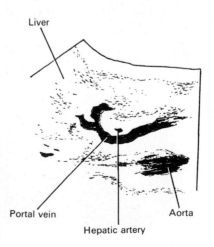

Liver

Portal vein

Hepatic artery

Aorta

F

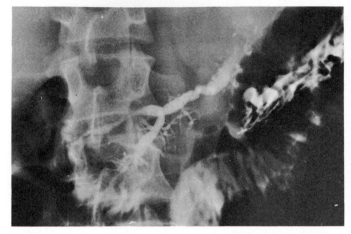

G

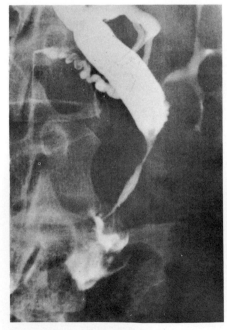

H

148

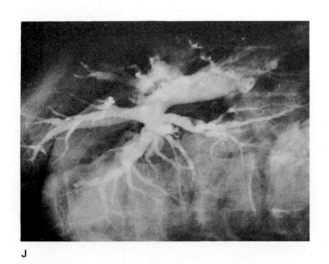

J

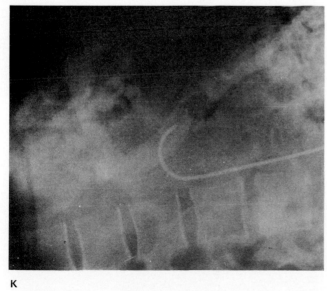

K

6.7 Acute hemorrhagic pancreatitis

This 58-year-old male teetotaler developed severe acute pancreatitis with drop in hematocrit and presented in shock, typical of acute hemorrhagic pancreatitis. He was referred to ultrasound for a baseline study since he was a strong candidate for the eventual development of a pseudocyst. It was also hoped that examination of the gallbladder might be able to establish an etiology.

An upper GI series (Fig. 6.7A) showed marked displacement of the stomach, duodenum and small bowel, typical of a markedly enlarged pancreas. An intra venous cholangiogram failed to give adequate visualization, but ultrasound demonstrated gallstones (Fig. 6.7B) as the cause of his pancreatitis.

A transverse echogram (Fig. 6.7C) of this very large patient shows a large, ill-defined prevertebral mass, consistent with marked enlargement of the pancreas. A sagittal section over the aorta, demonstrating the superior mesenteric artery and a branch of the celiac trunk, shows marked irregular enlargement of the pancreas, appearances consistent with an acute phlegmon.

The patient was scanned weekly to monitor the resolution of his pancreatitis. However, after a two-week interval, he presented with a markedly enlarged necrotic pancreas with areas of cystic formation in the body and tail of the pancreas. Comparison of the transverse and sagittal sections (Figs. 6.7E and 6.7F) demonstrates marked pancreatic enlargement with cystic formation, indicating a developing pseudocyst. Because of his stormy clinical course, surgery was performed and a pseudocyst with friable walls was drained into the stomach.

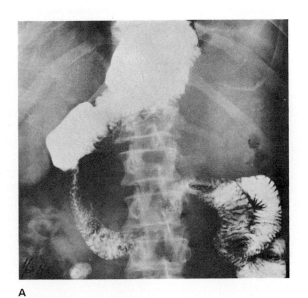

A

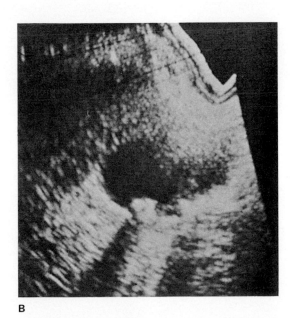

B

151

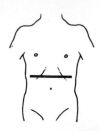

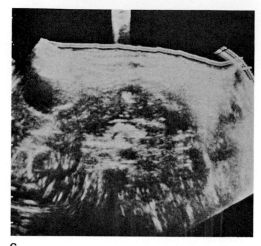

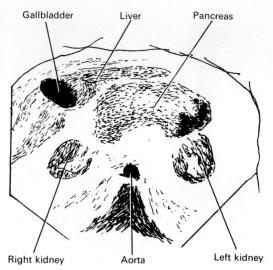

Gallbladder   Liver   Pancreas

Right kidney   Aorta   Left kidney

C

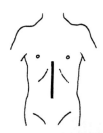

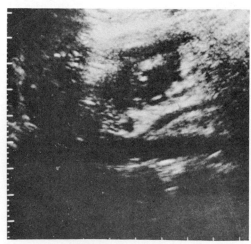

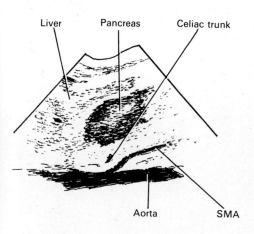

Liver   Pancreas   Celiac trunk

Aorta   SMA

D

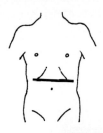

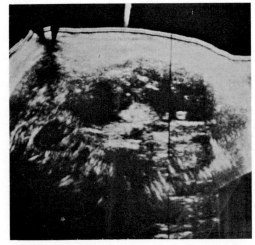

E

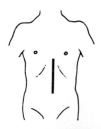

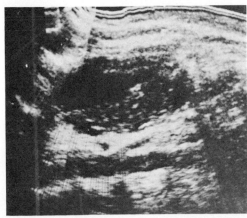

F

153

6.8 Pseudocyst

A middle-aged chronic alcoholic presented with a normal serum amylase and an enlarging mass in the epigastrium. A sagittal section (Fig. 6.8A) over the inferior vena cava reveals a large cystic mass just caudal to the portal vein. A second sagittal section (Fig. 6.8B) above the aorta demonstrates the superior mesenteric vein and the splenic artery with an ill-defined mass in the body of the pancreas. Transverse section (Fig. 6.8C) shows a large pseudocyst in the head of the pancreas juxtaposed to the gallbladder. It is important in diagnosing pseudocysts of the head of the pancreas to locate the gallbladder to avoid a mistaken identity. A second transverse section (Fig. 6.8D) slightly more cephalad reveals the body and tail of the pancreas above the superior mesenteric vessels. Transverse and sagittal sections (Fig. 6.8E and F) from a follow-up examination two months later demonstrate a decrease in the size of the pseudocyst.

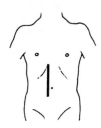

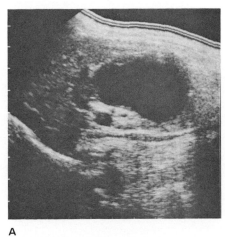

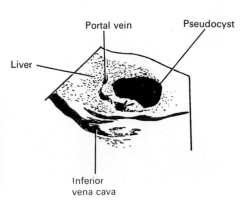

Portal vein   Pseudocyst

Liver

Inferior
vena cava

A

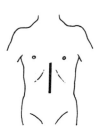

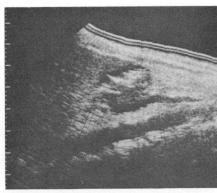

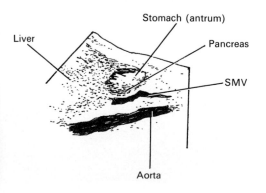

Stomach (antrum)

Pancreas

Liver

SMV

Aorta

B

155

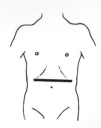

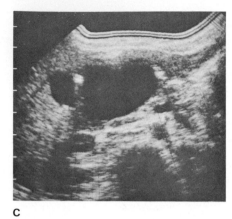

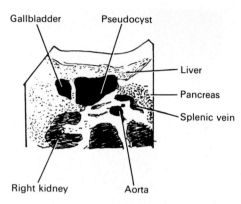

Gallbladder   Pseudocyst

Liver

Pancreas

Splenic vein

Right kidney   Aorta

C

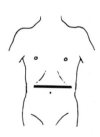

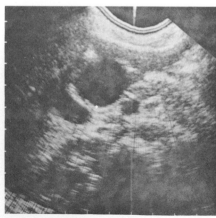

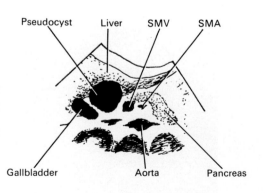

Pseudocyst   Liver   SMV   SMA

Gallbladder   Aorta   Pancreas

D

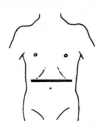

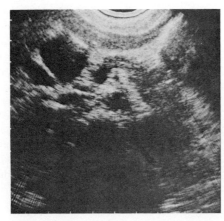

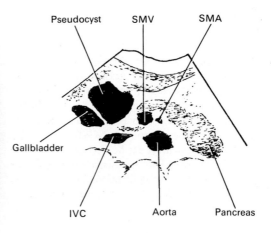

Pseudocyst   SMV   SMA

Gallbladder

IVC   Aorta   Pancreas

E

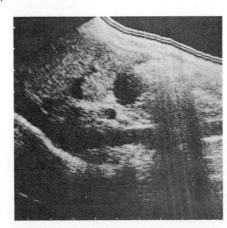

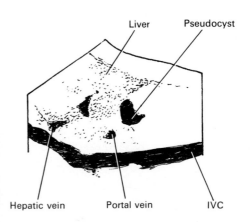

Liver   Pseudocyst

Hepatic vein   Portal vein   IVC

F

6.9 Pseudocyst

This 27-year-old chronic male alcoholic presented with an epigastric mass and an elevated serum amylase. A transverse scan (Fig. 6.9A) demonstrated a cystic mass in the prevertebral region. On the sagittal scan (Fig. 6.9B) above the aorta this cystic mass lies posterior to the liver and cephalad to the celiac trunk, thus localizing it in the lesser sac, a not uncommon location for pseudocyst formation. The ill-defined pancreas is noted between the superior mesenteric artery and the left lobe of the liver with its cephalad limit at the vertically oriented celiac trunk. The patient was aggressively treated with medical therapy for a two-week period. He was then allowed to eat and within 24 hours developed severe epigastric pain. The second examination (Fig. 6.9C and D) showed enlargement of the pseudocyst with the development of multiple internal echoes indicative of necrotic debris. There was no drop in hematocrit to indicate hemorrhage. On this examination there is a suggestion that the wall is becoming thicker, thus indicating that the pseudocyst is maturing.

Aggressive medical therapy was reinstituted and a reexamination in two weeks demonstrated a decrease in size of the pseudocyst with disappearance of the previously noted necrotic debris. Two weeks after this study the pseudocyst disappeared without symptoms, presumably by spontaneous drainage.

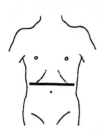

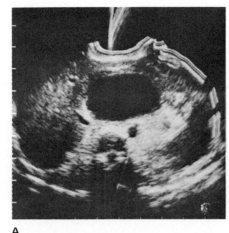

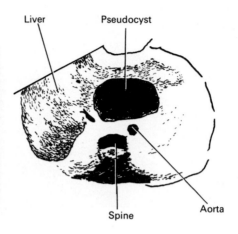

A

Liver   Pseudocyst

Spine   Aorta

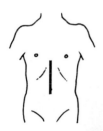

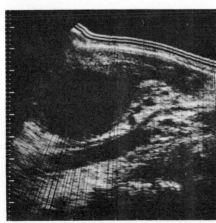

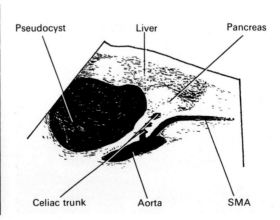

B

Pseudocyst   Liver   Pancreas

Celiac trunk   Aorta   SMA

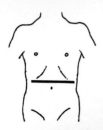

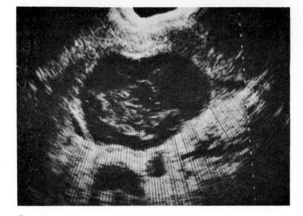

C

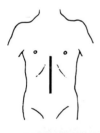

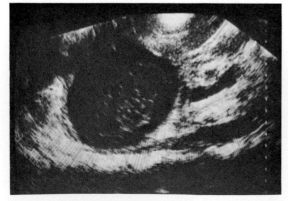

D

160

6.10 Pancreatic pseudocyst

This 24-year-old black male presented with a three-week history of abdominal pain, elevated serum amylase, and a palpable left upper quadrant mass. A previous history of pancreatitis was also elicited. Transverse section (A) of the left upper quadrant reveals a predominantly cystic mass with irregular walls and multiple internal echoes in its posterior region. Note the marked anterior and medial displacement of the left kidney which is flattened and rests anterior to the spine. A longitudinal section (B) in decubitus position shows the solid tissue which has irregular margins and is heterogeneous, suggesting necrosis. There is a strong suggestion of a thick medial wall on both sections. These images are consistent with a predominantly cystic mass with necrosis and would be compatible with a necrotic tumor, organizing hematoma or pancreatic pseudocyst. The surgical exploration revealed a thick walled, encapsulated pseudocyst of the tail of the pancreas with a marked amount of necrosis and cellular debris within it.

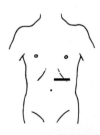

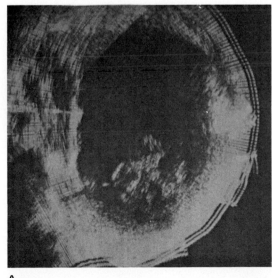

A

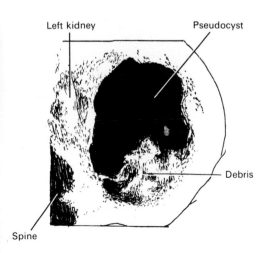

Left kidney

Pseudocyst

Debris

Spine

161

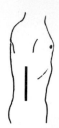

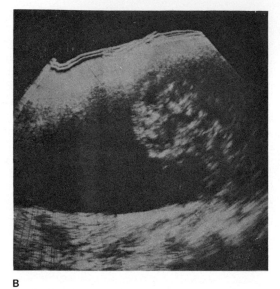

B

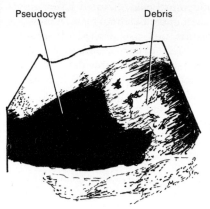

(Head) Right lateral decubitus (feet)

6.11 Carcinoma of head of pancreas

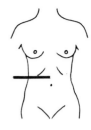

A 60-year-old patient was admitted for investigation of weight loss and penetrating back pain. There was no jaundice. A transverse ultrasonogram shows no evidence of biliary dilatation and the gallbladder is of normal size. In the prevertebral region, there is an irregular solid mass which is consistent with a carcinoma of the head of the pancreas. Approximately half of our patients at the present time are now diagnosed with carcinoma of the head of the pancreas before the onset of obstructive jaundice. In this patient, the diagnosis was confirmed with computerized axial tomograph (CAT) and the patient underwent surgery confirming both the ultrasound and CT findings. Unfortunately a complete resection was not possible.

Percutaneous biopsy of the pancreas may be helpful in such a patient and can be carried out under ultrasonic guidance. Over 1200 have been performed in Copenhagen with only four minor complications and no mortality (Rasmussen, personal communication). This appears to be a technique with great promise for the future, especially when high resolution, real-time scanners enable the procedure to be performed under "ultrasonic fluoroscopy."

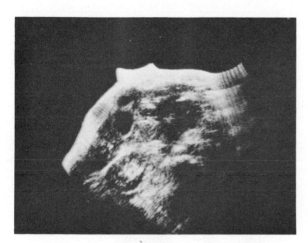

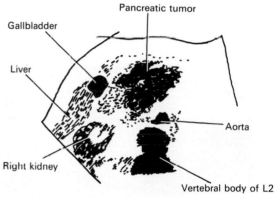

6.12 Carcinoma of the head with biliary obstruction

A 55-year-old male entered with weight loss and painless jaundice. A transverse echogram (A) reveals a large, homogeneous, ill-defined mass in the head of the pancreas and a dilated gallbladder with layering of sediment. A sagittal scan (B) above the inferior vena cava demonstrates the portal vein and a dilated common duct coursing inferiorly to the large mass in the head of the pancreas. Also noted are dilated intrahepatic biliary ducts in the liver. A second sagittal section (C) in the right lobe of the liver shows a dilated intrahepatic biliary tree as well as the obstructed gallbladder with sediment. Sediment in the gallbladder is often the result of bile stasis secondary to an obstructing common duct lesion and does not necessarily represent a diseased gallbladder. Operation revealed an unresectable carcinoma in the head of the pancreas.

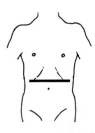

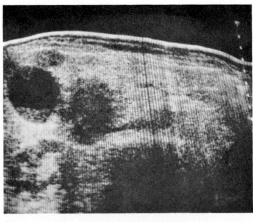

A

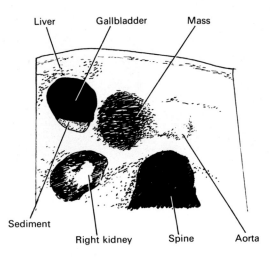

Liver Gallbladder Mass

Sediment

Right kidney Spine Aorta

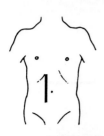

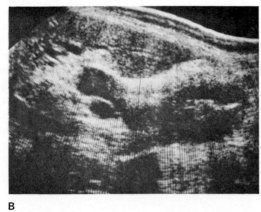

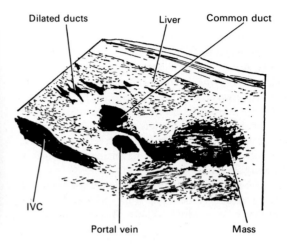

Dilated ducts   Liver   Common duct

IVC

Portal vein   Mass

B

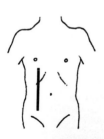

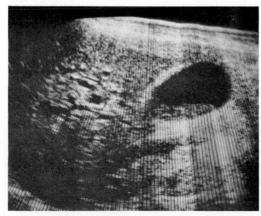

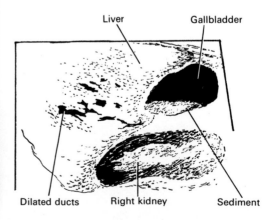

Liver   Gallbladder

Dilated ducts   Right kidney   Sediment

C

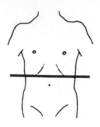

6.13 Carcinoma

A 60-year-old male with a history of weight loss and back pain presented for ultrasonic examination of the pancreas. A transverse echogram shows the splenic vein coursing across the midline anterior to the superior mesenteric artery. The high-level echoes between the splenic vein and the liver represent a region of the neck of the pancreas. Just to the left of the splenic vein is an ill-defined, irregular solid mass which returns low-level echoes and represents a carcinoma arising at the junction of the body and tail of the pancreas.

Just to the left of the liver there is a marked amount of scattering and reverberation from the overlying air-containing bowel which makes this region of the pancreas, the junction of the body and tail, the most difficult to visualize. However, additional techniques may be helpful. With the patient prone, scans through the acoustic window provided by the left kidney are used to visualize the tail of the pancreas. In decubitus positions movement of the liver and spleen may displace bowel gas and provide an acoustic window to the pancreas. Occasionally filling the stomach with fluid may be helpful. It is in this particular region that the CAT scanning may be valuable. However, in this patient who was thin, the pancreas was poorly outlined by CAT, a problem often ecountered in patients with abdominal neoplasms and marked weight loss.

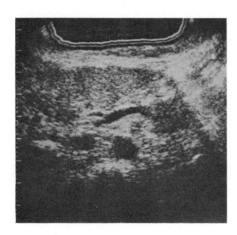

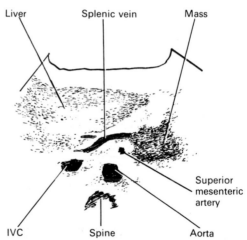

6.14 Carcinoma of the body

This 57-year-old female was admitted with a three-month history of abdominal pain, anorexia and weight loss. Because of the strong clinical suspicion for a pancreatic lesion, an echogram was performed. The two scans on this page are parasagittal sections of the aorta which show an ill-defined mass just anterior to the origin of the superior mesenteric artery. A transverse scan (p. 168) in the same region demonstrates a 2.5 cm localized mass lying immediately anterior to the superior mesenteric artery and beneath the left lobe of the liver. The superior mesenteric vein is seen slightly to the right. Knowing the exact location of the pancreas in relation to the mesenteric vessels permitted a correct diagnosis of primary carcinoma of the pancreas. An ERCP demonstrated complete obstruction of the main pancreatic duct. At surgery a successful radical resection was performed.

Confusion often arises as to whether a localized mass in the pancreatic region is of pancreatic origin or represents a metastasis. In general, nodes are located along the great vessels and, when enlarged, displace the mesenteric vessels anteriorly, producing a mass between the mesenteric vessels and the aorta. However, a mass anterior to the mesenteric vessels is, most likely, primarily pancreatic in origin since this is the space the pancreas occupies. Thus, using the mesenteric vessels as a dividing landmark the etiology of a solitary mass in this region may be determined with great regularity. Likewise the splenic vein acts as a similar landmark in the body and tail of the pancreas.

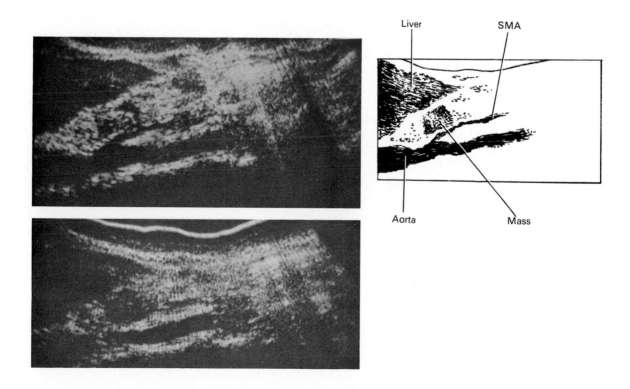

Liver   SMA

Aorta   Mass

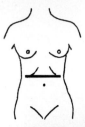

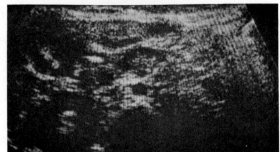

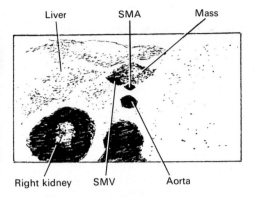

Liver   SMA   Mass

Right kidney   SMV   Aorta

Conclusion

Ultrasound has currently assumed an important role in the diagnosis of pancreatic disease. With the advent of the gray scale technique and the recognition of tissue consistency, evaluation of pancreatic disease has become more specific. Diseases that affect the pancreas are limited in number and present images that can be readily differentiated. Because the ultrasound exam is noninvasive and can be repeated as necessary, it has a particular advantage in the rapidly changing course of inflammatory diseases of the pancreas. It is ideally suited for following the patient with pancreatitis who is at risk to develop a pseudocyst. Ultrasound may establish diagnosis of pancreatitis by detecting an enlarged pancreas in the presence of a normal amylase, thus explaining the etiology of a previous episode of pain. As yet echography has added little to the early detection of pancreatic neoplasm.

The ability of ultrasound to examine several organ systems simultaneously is of particular advantage in the pancreas since concomitant disease in the liver, gallbladder and biliary tree as well as changes in the spleen and portal system are often associated with pancreatic disease. At the same time symptom complexes which often simulate those of pancreatic disease may be found to be caused by extra pancreatic pathology. Masses in the epigastrium may be differentiated as to etiology.

The complementary use of computerized tomography is still being evaluated. CT scanning certainly seems to be advantageous in those obese patients with prominent fat and well-defined fascia planes, whereas ultrasound appears to provide better images in thin patients. Obviously, a combination of imaging modalities including nuclear medicine, angiography, CT scanning and ultrasound will lead to greater diagnostic specificity. However, the special features of improved resolution, safety, low cost and the ease of repeating an exam insure an important place for ultrasound in the examination of the pancreas.

7. The spleen

ULTRASOUND SCANNING OF THE SPLEEN

The spleen is a difficult organ to evaluate clinically owing to its concealed position under the left costal margin. Considerable enlargement must occur before it is clinically palpable, and even then clinical assessment of the consistency of the organ is of little diagnostic value. The spleen is imaged by a liver-spleen isotope scan using ^{99m}Technetium labeled sulphur colloid, but this merely shows space-occupying defects and an approximation of splenic size.

Ultrasound has been used to estimate the volume of the spleen (Kardel, Holm, Rasmussen et al., 1971). The introduction of gray scale techniques, which resulted in the display of the normal tissue consistency, permits the possible differential diagnosis of splenomegaly based on the characteristic patterns of the splenic consistency (Taylor and Milan, 1976).

The spleen is a difficult organ to scan if it is of normal size and becomes progressively easier as the size increases. The normal-sized spleen must be scanned either obliquely along the tenth intercostal space or in the coronal plane in the midaxillary line. These techniques are considered at some length. The enlarged spleen may be examined by either technique, but in addition may be scanned by simple parasagittal scans like those used for the liver or by simple transverse scanning.

Oblique intercostal scans of the spleen

For the oblique intercostal scan of the spleen, the patient lies in the right lateral (decubitus) position. It is often helpful to abduct and fully extend the arm, which tends to widen the left intercostal spaces. Occasionally it may be necessary to use a pillow under the right side of the patient to further widen the left intercostal spaces. The costal margin is now identified in the region of the midaxillary line and the plane of the lowest intercostal space is defined. The skin is liberally smeared with oil and the transducer placed on the chest wall just anterior to the midaxillary line. The characteristic A-scan through the spleen is shown in Figure 7.1. It will be noted that there are very low-level echoes from the splenic consistency and a large distal echo from the capsule. The position of the scanning arm is adjusted to allow a scan along the intercostal space, and to maintain contact with the skin it may be necessary to angle the transducer cephalad. The spleen is now scanned along the tenth intercostal space (Fig. 7.2A); in this position, it will be found that the spleen is surprisingly anterior, lying between the midaxillary line and the left anterior subcostal margin. If the spleen is not satisfactorily imaged in this intercostal space, a higher intercostal space should be used. The advantage of this scan is that the longitudinal axis of the spleen lies along the intercostal space, so that scans of this axis allow us to quantitate the splenic size. A resulting scan is shown in Figure 7.2B. In these scans, it is frequently necessary to compound to outline the entire spleen. The echo amplitude is still apparent despite the degradation of resolution inherent in the use of compounding techniques (p. 9). The alternative scanning method to this oblique intercostal scan is the longitudinal scan in the coronal plane.

Longitudinal coronal scan of the spleen

Again the patient is scanned in the right lateral (decubitus) position. The mechanical scanning arm is arranged so that it is in line with the patient's body and the lower intercostal spaces are identified in the midaxillary line. The skin is again liberally smeared with paraffin oil and small sector movements are made in the lowest intercostal space which may be palpated. These scans are carried out in deep inspiration, since this rotates the lower ribs and increases the size of the intercostal spaces. Extreme rotation of the transducer is required to write the left hemidiaphragm. This is shown schematically in Figure 7.3A. The spleen is seen as a highly homogeneous organ lying between the upper pole of the left kidney and the left hemidiaphragm. A spleen scan obtained by this technique is shown in Figure 7.3B.

Markedly enlarged spleens can be scanned in either the paramedian plane or in the transverse plane in a similar way to that described in Chapter 2 for liver scanning (p. 15). A paramedian scan of the spleen is shown in Figure 7.11 and a transverse scan is shown in Figure 7.8.

REFERENCES

Kardel, T., Holm, H.H., Rasmussen, S.N. and Mortensen, T.: Ultrasonic determination of liver and spleen volume. *Scand. J. Clin. and Lab. Invest.*, **27**, 123–128, 1971.

Taylor, K.J.W. and Milan, J.: Differential diagnosis of chronic splenomegaly by grey-scale ultrasonography: clinical observation and digital A-scan analysis. *Brit. J. Radiol.*, **49**, 519–525, 1976.

7.1 Ultrasound scanning of the spleen

An A-scan through an enlarged spleen shows very low-level echoes arising from within the organ; large echoes are seen proximally from the initial pulse and a larger distal echo is seen from the capsule of the spleen. It is important not to confuse these appearances with those due to fluid collections, such as left subphrenic abscesses.

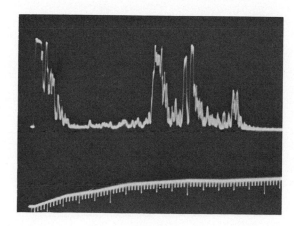

7.2 Ultrasound scanning of the spleen

A. Schema to show movement of the transducer to produce an oblique intercostal scan of the spleen. The transducer is placed in the tenth intercostal space and rocked in small arcs along the tenth interspace.

B. B-mode ultrasonogram of spleen produced by the oblique intercostal scanning method.

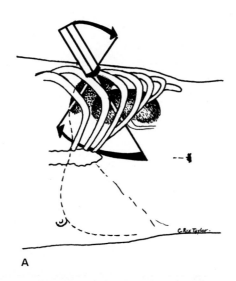

A

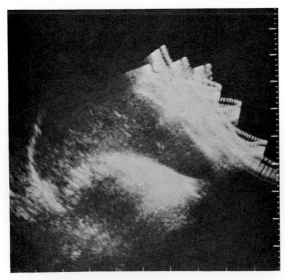

B

7.3 Ultrasound scanning of the spleen

A. Schema to show movement of the transducer to produce a longitudinal coronal scan of the spleen. The transducer is placed in the lower intercostal spaces in the midaxillary line and then moved through a simple arc in the coronal plane.

B. B-mode ultrasonogram of spleen produced by the longitudinal coronal scanning method.

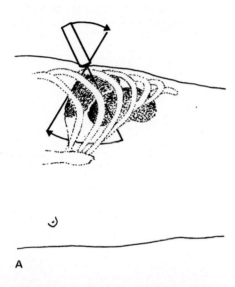

A

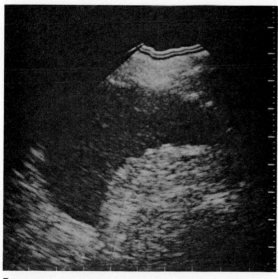

B

7.4 Traumatic splenic cyst

This 14-year-old boy was noted to have a left upper quadrant mass on routine physical examination. The pediatrician considered that this might be splenomegaly due to Gaucher's disease. The patient's brother had died of a malignant lymphoma only three months previously.

All fears of serious disease were allayed by this ultrasound examination. The transverse ultrasonogram of the trunk (above) shows a large echo-free area in the left upper quadrant, while the longitudinal ultrasono-gram (below) shows a large cystic cavity limited by the left hemidiaphragm above and compressed spleen posteriorly. The correct diagnosis of a simple splenic cyst was made immediately. Subsequent investigation by intravenous pyelography revealed a normal left kidney except for inferior displacement, while an isotopic liver-spleen scan showed a large splenic defect. At eventual surgery, the presence of a splenic cyst was confirmed.

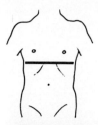

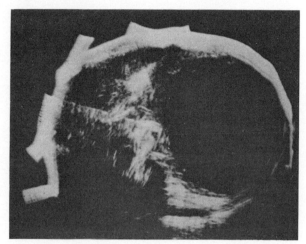

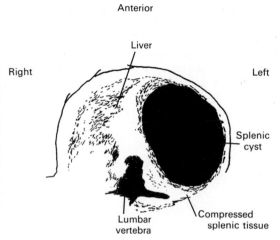

Anterior

Liver

Right

Left

Splenic
cyst

Lumbar
vertebra

Compressed
splenic tissue

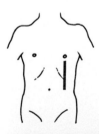

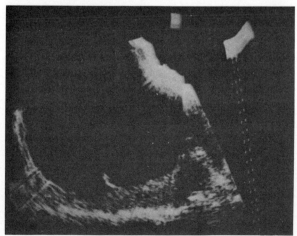

7.5 Traumatic splenic cyst

This 12-year-old boy presented with a large palpable left upper quadrant mass and a history of previous injury to that site.

A longitudinal sector scan in the left parasagittal plane (upper figure) shows a large, echo-free area lying anterior to the left kidney with a rim of compressed splenic tissue around the cyst.

These appearances are confirmed on the transverse scan with the patient in the decubitus position (lower figure). Again, a compressed spleen is seen between the upper pole of the left kidney and the cyst.

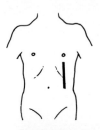

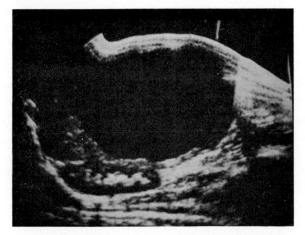

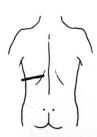

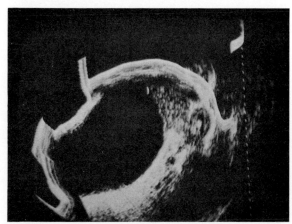

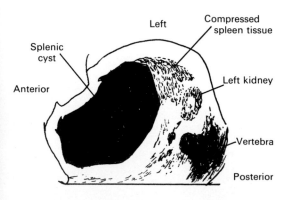

Anterior

Splenic
cyst

Left

Compressed
spleen tissue

Left kidney

Vertebra

Posterior

7.6 Traumatic hematoma

This 24-year-old female was noted to have a left upper quadrant mass when admitted in labor. After delivery the mass was investigated. The transverse ultrasonogram (above) reveals a mass lying anterior to the spleen but apparently possessing a similar structure to the spleen. The longitudinal ultrasonogram (below) shows a uniform mass lying between the upper pole of the left kidney and the compressed spleen. The differential diagnosis included a suprarenal tumor, a retroperitoneal lymphoma, and an organizing splenic hematoma. An isotope scan revealed a large splenic defect, intravenous pyelography showed displacement of the left kidney downwards, and CT scanning confirmed the presence of a solid left upper quadrant mass. Surgery was delayed for approximately six weeks and revealed a splenic cyst with changed blood in its walls, indicating its origin from a hematoma.

There appears to be no doubt that this was an organizing hematoma at the time of the investigation, which resulted in a cyst after further organization of the clot. Undue delay between an ultrasound examination and surgery may result in apparent discrepancies and the sceptical surgeon may not appreciate that change has occurred. Repeat examination immediately before surgery in this patient would have demonstrated the then-fluid contents and modified the surgical incision.

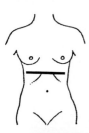

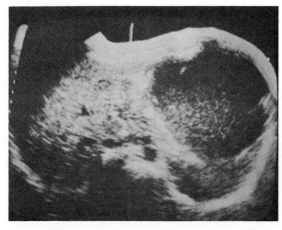

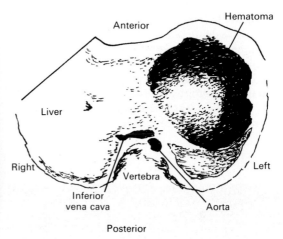

Anterior

Hematoma

Liver

Right

Left

Vertebra

Inferior
vena cava

Aorta

Posterior

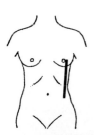

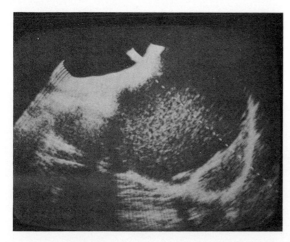

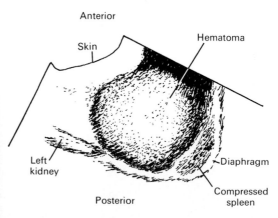

Anterior

Skin

Hematoma

Left
kidney

Diaphragm

Compressed
spleen

Posterior

179

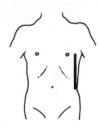

7.7 Splenomegaly due to portal hypertension

This patient was referred for ultrasonic examination due to progressive development of jaundice. On ultrasound examination of the liver, obvious cirrhosis was present with enlargement and tortuosity of the portal vein, similar to the appearances seen in Figure 4.36. With the patient in the decubitus position, a longitudinal coronal scan of the spleen was carried out; it is shown in the ultrasonogram. The splenic vessels usually divide into a number of branches prior to entering the hilum of the spleen, and the splenic vessels are seen in this scan. The spleen is limited by apposition with the chest wall anteriorly and by the dome of the left hemidiaphragm posteriorly. Splenic consistency is characteristic of congestive splenomegaly and reveals medium-level echoes distributed in a fine and uniform pattern.

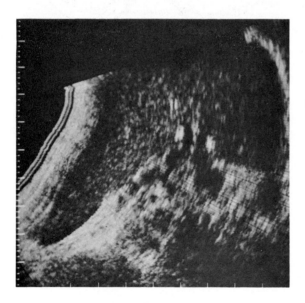

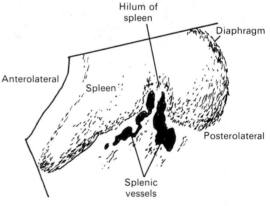

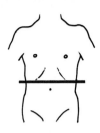

7.8 Benign enlargement in nontropical hepatosplenomegaly

An 80-year-old male presented with palpable hepatosplenomegaly discovered during routine clinical examination. Clinically he was considered to have a malignancy. The ultrasonogram is a transverse section through the spleen and shows a definite pattern. The echo amplitude is not in the very low range found in both normal and malignant spleens. Most untreated malignant spleens appear very black, although the precise appearance will vary with the signal-to-noise ratio of any given machine. Gray scale techniques are an essential prerequisite to the differential diagnosis of splenomegaly by ultrasound.

This patient was intensely investigated but no evidence of malignancy was found. His final diagnosis was nontropical hepatosplenomegaly.

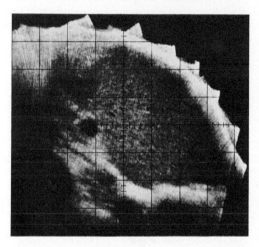

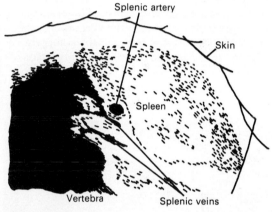

Transverse section of abdomen in left subcostal region

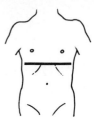

7.9 Chronic inflammatory state

This middle-aged male, a Libyan, presented with malaise and fever. Examination revealed lymphadenopathy and hepatosplenomegaly. The provisional diagnosis was a lymphoma. Transverse ultrasonic examination revealed the tip of the liver, which returns very high-level echoes, and marked splenomegaly, also with very high internal echoes. The left and right kidneys and psoas major muscles are well seen posteriorly.

High-level echoes are seldom seen in untreated malignancy of the spleen, while untreated lymphomatous infiltration of the liver has never been reported or noted to produce high-level echoes. This examination was therefore at variance with the clinical impression and suggests that the cause of hepatosplenomegaly was more likely to be a chronic inflammatory state. At surgery, white nodules were found throughout the spleen at splenectomy; and similar findings were apparent on a wedge biopsy of the liver. Macroscopically, malignancy was still simulated. The eventual histology proved it to be tuberculosis and no evidence of any malignant state was found. This patient was subsequently successfully treated with antituberculous therapy.

This case, which occurred early in 1973 during the clinical evaluation of the gray scale technique, demonstrates the unique information which may be available to the ultrasonographer which at times allows him to successfully challenge the apparent clinical and surgical impressions.

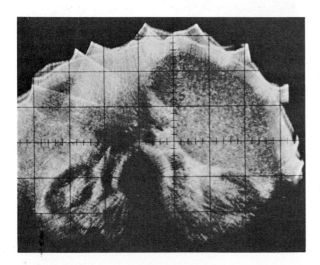

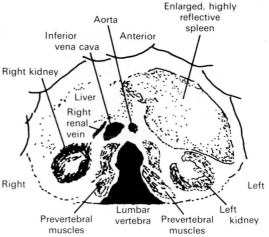

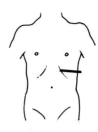

7.10 Metastatic involvement

Metastatic involvement of the spleen is rare but occurred in this elderly male with a carcinoma of the colon and marked metastatic involvement of the liver on initial presentation. This oblique ultrasonogram along the 10th intercostal space shows enlargement of the spleen and several highly echogenic masses within it. The liver metastases were also echogenic. In this patient, metastatic involvement of the spleen from the colon may have been facilitated by the massive liver involvement, producing portal vein obstruction and reversed flow in the portal vein.

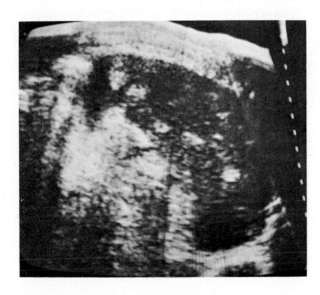

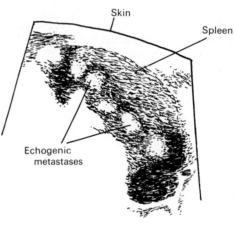

7.11 Chronic myeloid leukemia

This 66-year-old patient was referred for evaluation of the spleen. She was known to suffer from chronic myeloid leukemia and had been extensively treated for the past two years.

A transverse ultrasonogram (upper figure) using a compounded technique to produce an axial tomogram shows a large, highly homogeneous organ which fills the left hypochondrium and extends over the midline into the right hypochondrium. Note that very low-level echoes are seen from within this mass, although the TGC brings out fine echoes in the deeper parts of the massively enlarged spleen.

A longitudinal ultrasonogram using a simple sector scan in the parasagittal plane again reveals marked enlargement of the spleen, which extends inferiorly as far as the umbilicus. Again, the organ is seen to be highly homogeneous although the TGC brings out a fine pattern in the deeper parts of the spleen.

The amplitude of the echoes from within the splenic consistency will vary according to the amount of signal-to-noise ratio in the individual diagnostic equipment, including the characteristics of the transducer in use at that time. However, under standard conditions it has been noted that acute malignancy in the spleen tends to return very low-level echoes and appears almost cystic. These appearances may change with prolonged therapy, resulting in high-level echoes. The appearances in congestive splenomegaly show intermediate-level echoes, while very high-level echoes are predominantly found in chronic inflammatory states. This variation in amplitude of the returned echoes is similar to that found in chronic inflammatory states affecting the liver.

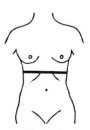

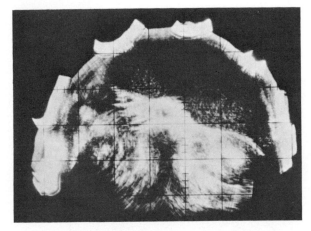

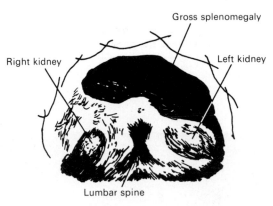

Gross splenomegaly

Right kidney

Left kidney

Lumbar spine

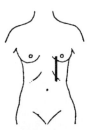

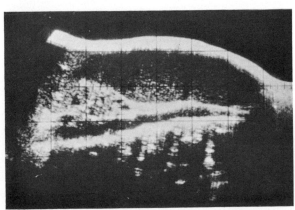

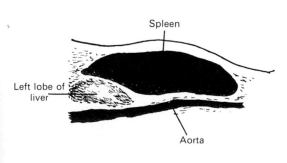

Spleen

Left lobe of liver

Aorta

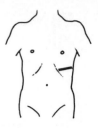

7.12 Infarct due to bacterial endocarditis

A 22-year-old male with congenital aortic stenosis presented with acute bacterial endocarditis and signs of peripheral emboli. He was referred for ultrasonic examination to investigate the possibility of other septic foci.

A longitudinal scan through the spleen in the midaxillary line shows definite splenic enlargement with a highly reflective mass just below the left hemidiaphragm. These appearances suggest a mass of fibrous tissue and are consistent with a splenic infarct associated with his bacterial endocarditis.

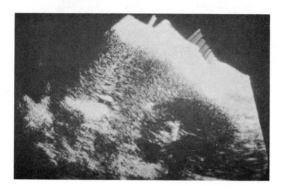
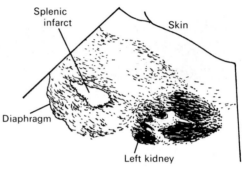

8. The kidney

NEPHROSONOGRAPHY

Introduction

Gray scale ultrasound offers a safe and rapid means to image the kidneys, perirenal region, ureters, and bladder. The information obtained complements that available from other imaging modalities. Renal size can be assessed in three dimensions. Parenchymal lesions can be identified and differentiated into those with cystic and those with solid consistencies. In addition, the liver is routinely examined and the presence or absence of hepatic metastases, cysts, and fibrosis can be determined (p. 226). The combination of renal and hepatic ultrasound imaging may permit a diagnosis which could not otherwise be made by noninvasive modalities.

The right kidney is initially scanned through the liver. The study is made during suspended, deep inspiration with a single pass, as described by Taylor and Hill (1974). The transducer is moved in an arc to encompass the right kidney and liver. Figure 8.1 (p. 189) shows the resulting scan. The characteristic internal architecture of the liver is seen and there are lower level echoes within the parenchyma of the kidney. The collecting system is noted as a central zone of higher level echoes. With the patient prone, each kidney can be scanned longitudinally and transversely (Fig. 8.3, p. 192). The normal ureter is not usually identified. Sector scans from the lateral aspect with the patient supine permit additional transverse scans to be written with high resolution. On occasion the decubitus position or the upright position may permit the identification of a lesion which cannot be seen in the routine projection. The highest frequency transducer which will penetrate the patient should be used for optimum resolution.

8.1 Normal anatomy

A. Figure 8.1A demonstrates a longitudinal parasagittal section through the liver and right kidney of a 5-year-old. Note the homogeneous echo pattern within the normal liver parenchyma. The right kidney is seen with a central collection of high level echoes representing the collecting system. The cortex has an echo pattern which is of a lower level than that of the liver and collecting system. Projections of the cortex (septa or columns of Bertin) are seen radiating toward the central collecting system. The medulla appears as a relatively echo-free zone. This appearance of the medulla should not be mistaken for cysts or other pathology. The arcuate vessels are represented by punctate echoes at the corticomedullary junction. Delineation of the actual structure of the parenchyma of the kidney permits the identification of relatively small lesions less than 1 cm in size when they are within the cortex. In addition, cortical thickness can be evaluated. This scan was obtained with a single pass in suspended respiration at a relatively high gain. (See Cook, Rosenfield and Taylor, 1977.)

B. This figure shows a transverse section of the right kidney in the same patient, obtained with the patient supine. The liver with its normal echo pattern is seen anteriorly. The kidney is relatively round in its transverse dimensions and the collecting system is seen as a zone of higher level echoes in the medial aspect of the kidney. Once again, the normal cortex and medulla can be differentiated. The renal artery and renal vein are seen in the renal hilum.

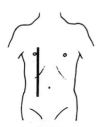

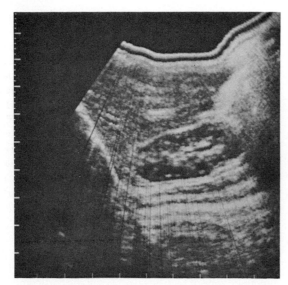

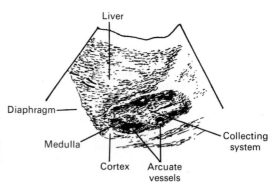

Liver

Diaphragm

Medulla

Cortex

Arcuate vessels

Collecting system

A

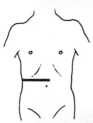

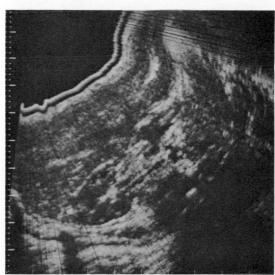

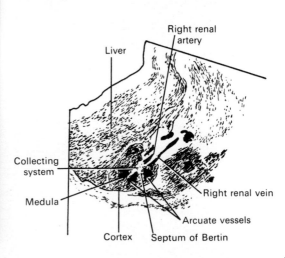

Right renal artery

Liver

Collecting system

Medula

Cortex

Septum of Bertin

Arcuate vessels

Right renal vein

B

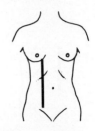

8.2 Normal anatomy—comparison of bistable and gray scale ultrasonography in the examination of the kidney

These longitudinal parasagittal sections through the liver and right kidney demonstrate the difference between the examination of the renal parenchyma with gray scale ultrasonography as it is currently used and the previous techniques that involved bistable machinery.

A. This figure shows a typical bistable scan through the liver and right kidney. The liver is seen to be relatively echo-free, and the right kidney has echo-free parenchyma with central echoes, representing the collecting system.

B. A high gain bistable examination of the liver and right kidney is seen. There are echoes in the liver. The parenchyma of the right kidney remains relatively sonolucent.

C. This figure demonstrates a longitudinal parasagittal scan through the liver and the right kidney of the same patient as in A and B. There is a characteristic echo pattern to the liver which is homogeneous with a few sonolucent zones, representing hepatic veins. The right kidney again can be seen with central echoes from the collecting system. In addition, the cortex appears as a more echogenic region than the medulla, which is relatively sonolucent. Compared to bistable equipment, gray scale ultrasonography involves better signal-to-noise ratio and improved resolution. The ability to appreciate the normal cortical echo pattern permits the identification of significantly smaller lesions than could previously be appreciated using bistable equipment. Note that the cortical echoes are lower in intensity than the central echoes from the pelvocalyceal system. With the deposition of collagen in the cortex—such as with diabetic glomerulosclerosis (Fig. 8.29)—the intensity of these echoes will be higher. In addition, in patients with transplant rejection the intensity of the echoes in the cortex may be exaggerated (p. 241). Optimal delineation of the renal cortex is obtained in thin patients when a relatively high frequency transducer can be used.

As noted in Figure 8.1 and above, an additional feature of gray scale ultrasound is that, in some patients, it permits the identification of the arcuate vessels as a punctuate zone of high-level echoes at the corticomedullary junction. These echoes in the region of the arcuate arteries serve as a marker to evaluate cortical thickness.

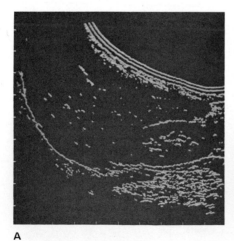

A

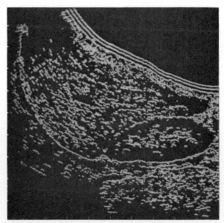

B

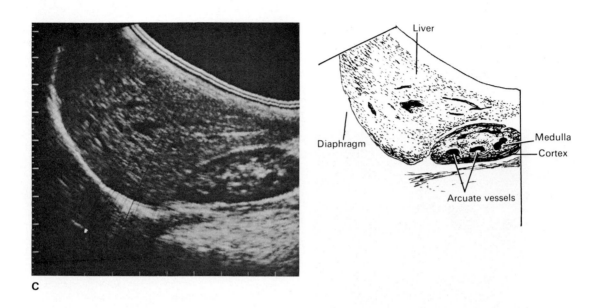

C

Liver

Diaphragm

Medulla

Cortex

Arcuate vessels

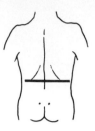

8.3 Normal anatomy—transverse scan with the patient prone

With the patient prone both kidneys can be written transversely, as shown here, and longitudinally. The collecting system is seen as an echogenic zone in the medial portion of each kidney. The best detail of the kidney is obtained when each one is sectioned individually, however, and this should also be routinely done.

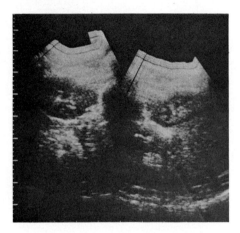
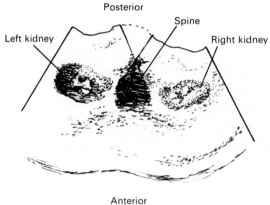

8.4 Normal anatomy—shadowing by gallstones

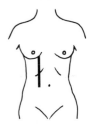

This longitudinal parasagittal section through the liver and right kidney demonstrates a gallstone within the gallbladder. The shadow behind the gallstone obscures a portion of the right kidney. The intimate relationship between the gallbladder and right kidney should be appreciated so that the effect of gallbladder disease upon the kidney will not be mistaken for renal pathology.

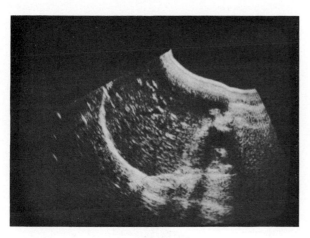

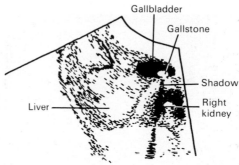

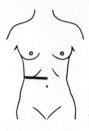

8.5 Normal anatomy—the right renal vein

The kidney is seen here in transverse section imaged from the anterior abdomen through the liver. The right renal vein is appreciated as a linear, echo-free structure running from the right kidney to the inferior vena cava. To the left of the inferior vena cava is the aorta, and the spine is seen behind the two great vessels. The right renal vein is routinely imaged but, because of differences in angulation, its actual size cannot be accurately ascertained. Occasionally it cannot be identified in normal patients, and the failure to find it during an ultrasonographic study cannot be used as an indication of renal vein pathology.

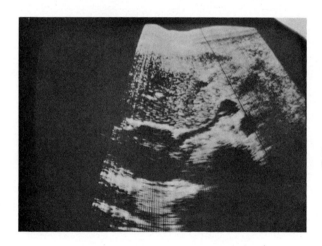

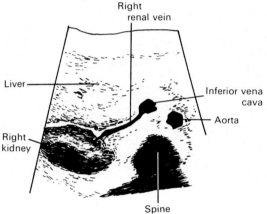

8.6 Normal anatomy—the left renal vein

The left renal vein is the only vascular structure to run between the superior mesenteric artery and aorta on transverse scanning. Also appreciated on this transverse scan is a portion of the pancreas. The inferior vena cava is collapsed.

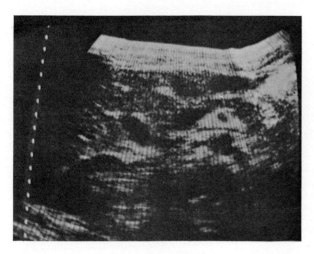

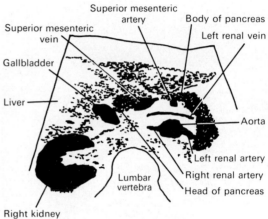

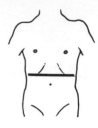

8.7 Normal anatomy—the renal arteries

A transverse scan demonstrates both kidneys. The renal arteries extend from the aorta, which is seen just left of the midline, to the kidneys. Behind the aorta is the spine.

The superior mesenteric artery is just anterior to the aorta. The inferior vena cava is collapsed and is not seen.

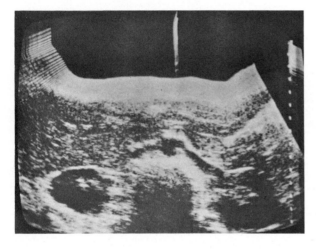

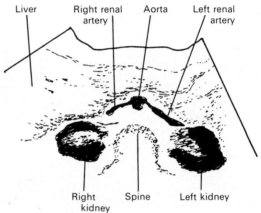

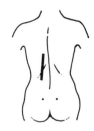

8.8 Congenital anomaly—duplication of the collecting system

A. This figure demonstrates a longitudinal section through the right kidney of a 24-year-old woman in the prone position. There are two separate central echoes seen, with an echo-free zone separating them. These two separate central echoes represent a duplex system in the right kidney of this patient. In contrast to hydronephrosis, each of these two central echoes is well formed and neither contains a separate central echo-free zone. Note that the anechoic area between the two collecting systems is not bordered on the superior margin by echoes, as would be expected if this represented a dilated renal pelvis.

B. An excretory urogram on the same patient demonstrates a duplicated system on the right. There is no evidence of hydronephrosis or other renal pathology.

(Courtesy of Daniel Myerson, M.D., Griffin Hospital, Derby, Connecticut.)

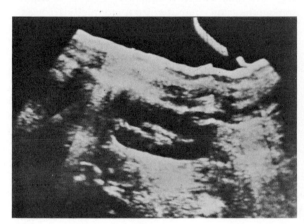

A

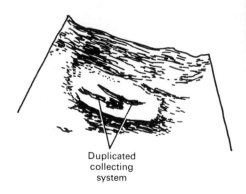

Duplicated
collecting
system

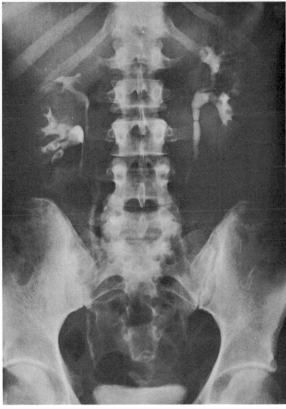

B

ULTRASOUND IN THE INVESTIGATION OF RENAL MASSES

Ultrasound is a standard modality for the investigation of renal masses and provides information which is complementary to other modalities in delineating the nature of a lesion which is present. The major role of ultrasound is in the differentiation of simple renal cysts from other processes such as tumor. The criteria for the diagnosis of a renal cyst are shown in Table 8.1.

Table 8.1

Renal cyst	Renal tumor
Echo-free	Internal echoes
Smooth walls	Irregular margins
Good transmission	Attenuation

A renal cyst is echo-free and has smooth walls. Because of the excellent transmission of the beam by the fluid in a cyst, there is little attenuation of the beam. The far wall echoes will, therefore, be equal to or, for technical reasons, higher than the near wall echo. This is an important criterion, since with the newer gray scale equipment a few low-level echoes representing noise may be seen in a simple renal cyst. Most renal tumors contain some echoes and attenuate the ultrasound beam. The far wall echoes, on A-mode, are generally lower in intensity than the near wall echoes. Occasional tumors,

particularly Wilms' tumor in childhood, may be relatively transsonic, mimicking a cystic lesion. We now feel, in fact, that a renal mass in childhood which by palpation feels solid and by ultrasound appears cystic is a Wilms' tumor.

The approach to renal masses used at the Yale–New Haven Hospital is shown in Table 8.2. A renal mass is generally first noted at urography. If the ultrasound examination indicates that the mass is a cyst, a cyst puncture is used to verify that one is not dealing with a cystic tumor or abscess. If the ultrasound indicates that there is a solid lesion, angiography is useful to delineate the blood supply to the tumor and to identify non-neoplastic lesions such as abscesses. On occasion, a lesion that appears solid on ultrasound can appear cystic at angiography. In this situation, cyst puncture or evaluation with computerized tomography will be of further aid in evaluating the lesion. When the ultrasound examination is equivocal, high dose nephrotomography and computerized tomography are used to evaluate the lesion. The approach used for any given patient must be individualized. For example, if a patient is not a surgical candidate because of a medical problem, cyst puncture is probably not justified. If the lesion on excretory urography is suggestive of a septum of Bertin, a static radioisotope study will show activity in a septum of Bertin but no activity in other renal masses such as cysts and tumors. However, lesions must be over 1.5 cm in size to be appreciated on the radioisotope study.

Table 8.2 Evaluation of renal mass lesions

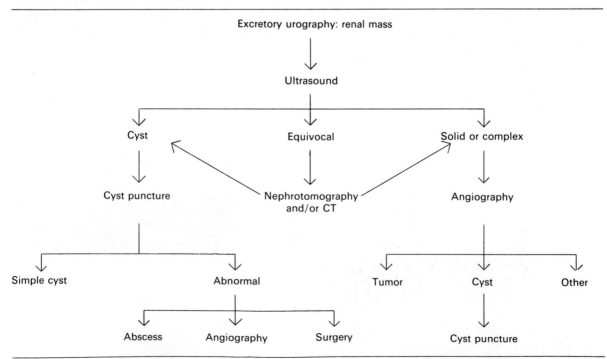

The technique of ultrasound scanning for the evaluation of renal mass lesions includes a single pass technique, suspended respiration, the demonstration of the lesion on A-mode and B-mode, and the use of the highest frequency transducer that will penetrate the patient. We perform our studies of renal masses at a single, relatively high gain which is adequate to produce echoes in the normal renal parenchyma.

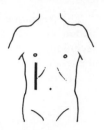

8.9 Renal masses—simple cyst

This elderly male presenting with hematuria had a mass in the upper pole of the right kidney demonstrated on excretory urography.

A. The longitudinal parasagittal section shown here demonstrates a normal lower pole to the right kidney and a $6\frac{1}{2}$ cm mass in the upper pole. The dot scale which is printed on the scan permits the ready measurement of the size of the lesion, with each interval equivalent to 1 cm. Note that on B-mode the lesion is echo-free, has smooth walls, and has high-level echoes forming its distal wall, indicating good transmission of the ultrasound beam. A portion of the liver is seen just above the mass.

B. On A-mode, the back wall of the lesion is seen to produce a significantly higher echo than on the front wall. This is due to better transmission of sound through homogeneous fluid than through solid tissue. There are a few very low-level echoes in the anterior portion of the cyst seen on A-mode, which represent reverberation artifact and should not be mistaken for internal echoes.

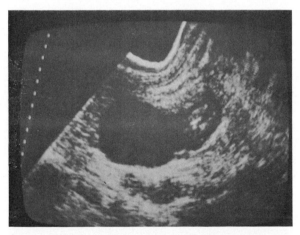

A

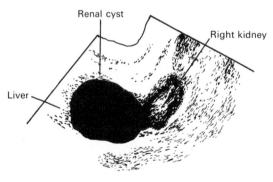

Renal cyst

Right kidney

Liver

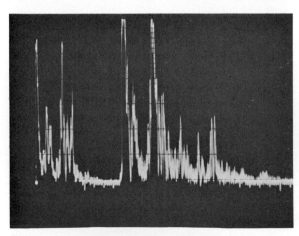

B

8.10 Renal masses—peripelvic cyst

This 58-year-old man presented with signs and symptoms of prostatic disease.

A. A routine excretory urogram demonstrates an abnormal axis and a mass medial to the left kidney.

B. Echo examination demonstrates an echo-free mass medial to the left kidney which, on B-mode, has the characteristics of a simple cyst. Note again the dot scale, with each interval between dots representing 1 cm.

C. A-mode also shows the characteristics of a simple cyst. The echoes at the back wall of the cyst are higher in level than the front wall echo.

At surgery for another problem, this was verified to be a simple renal cyst.

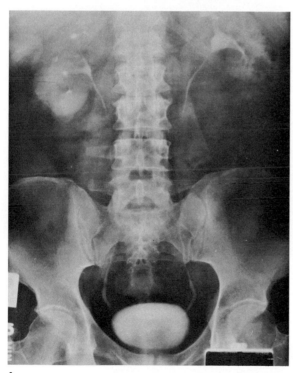

A

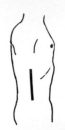

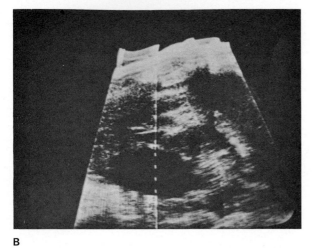

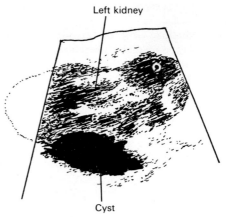

Left kidney

Cyst

B

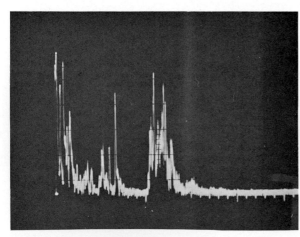

C

8.11 Renal masses—cyst puncture

A renal cyst is aspirated in the prone position under local anesthesia. Either fluoroscopy after an intravenous injection of contrast media or ultrasound guidance may be used. Ultrasound permits the depth of the lesion to be gauged and displays the needle tip in the cyst during the course of the procedure. The change in size of the cyst with respect to the position of the needle can be noted. The findings in a simple renal cyst at puncture are summarized in Table 8.3. A renal cyst should have clear or straw-colored fluid. Bloody fluid does not necessarily indicate a renal tumor, but only that this is not a simple renal cyst. For example, there may be hemorrhage into a renal cyst. Fluid should be withdrawn for cytology to exclude a renal tumor. If pus is obtained, it should be cultured. In addition, the lactic dehydrogenase (LDH)

in a simple renal cyst is typically less than blood level and renal cysts do not contain fat. Although contrast is frequently injected into renal cysts to evaluate the contour of the lesion under fluoroscopy, we do not believe this to be essential.

Table 8.3 Cyst puncture

Renal cyst	
Fluid	Clear
Cytology	Negative
LDH (lactic dehydrogenase)	Less than blood level
Fat	None

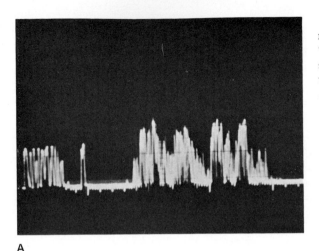

A

A. Renal cyst puncture under ultrasound guidance may involve the use of special transducers. A "doughnut"-shaped transducer produces an A-mode scan of the cyst. The needle, when it has been inserted through the hole in the doughnut, can be appreciated as a high level echo within the cyst, as this figure demonstrates. When the stylet is in place, the echo from the needle while it is in the cyst may not be appreciated. Therefore, the stylet should not be in place after one has entered the cyst.

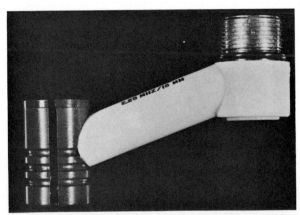

B

B. The alternative is the so-called "keyhole" transducer, with a side hole which permits removal of the transducer during the course of the study for use in B-mode imaging. In addition, this "keyhole" acts as an added safety factor should the patient or transducer be inadvertently moved.

The depth of the cyst should initially be noted on scanning prior to the puncture. This permits the choice of an appropriate needle length and also permits one to mark on the needle the depth to which one expects to go. In general, a small needle of approximately 20 gauge should be used to minimize the risk of the procedure. Complications are infrequent but include pneumothorax, hematuria, and infection.

An alternative method of renal cyst puncture under ultrasound guidance involves initial scanning in B-mode for the identification of the lesion. The cyst puncture is performed from the posterior aspect with the patient prone while scanning from the lateral aspect of the patient. The needle can be identified in the cyst and the size of the cyst can be observed on the B-mode as it is aspirated.

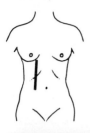

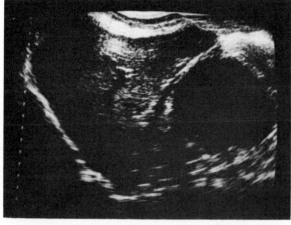

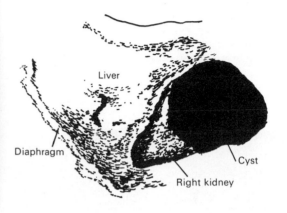

C

C. and D. These figures demonstrate the B-mode scans of a cyst before (C) and after (D) cyst puncture. Note that, although enough fluid has been withdrawn for evaluation, it is not necessary to aspirate the entire cyst. However, should a renal cyst be causing symptoms because of its size, the cyst can be aspirated and a sclerosing agent injected into it (Raskin, Poole, Roen, and Viamonte, 1975).

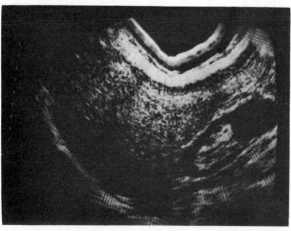

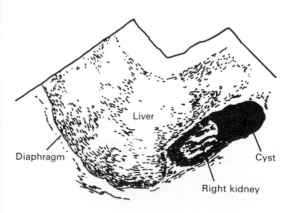

D

8.12 Renal masses—renal tumor

Longitudinal (A) and transverse (B) examination of the right kidney demonstrates an 11 cm mass extending from the lower pole of the kidney. The mass is clearly solid and contains internal echoes. There are focal zones that are echo-free, possibly representing tumor necrosis. In addition, on the transverse scan some localized calyceal dilatation can be seen. The border between the mass and the kidney is poorly defined, another finding which is consistent with tumor. At surgery a hypernephroma was found.

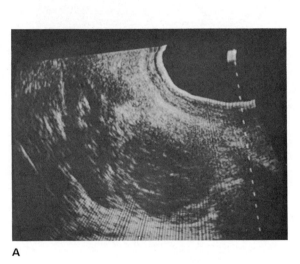

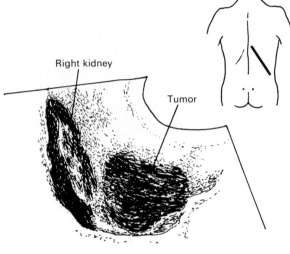

Right kidney

Tumor

A

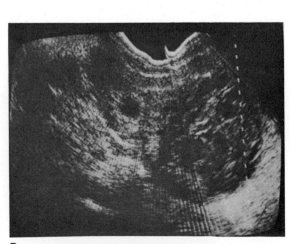

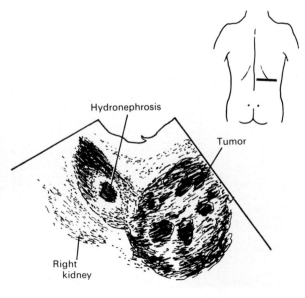

Hydronephrosis

Tumor

Right kidney

B

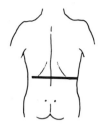

8.13 Renal masses—renal lymphoma

Lymphoma may involve one or both kidneys and may present as discrete masses or as infiltrative disease of the entire kidney. This 60-year-old male with known lymphoma presented with a right nonfunctioning kidney.

A. Ultrasound examination, in the transverse projection, demonstrates that the left kidney is replaced by an echo-producing mass. The lesion can be seen to have internal echoes. This indicates that it is solid and, when combined with the clinical history, would lead to the correct diagnosis of lymphoma involving the left kidney.

B. Here the A-mode demonstrates internal echoes within the lesion. There is good transmission, which is common with lymphoma.

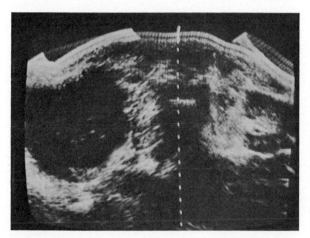

A

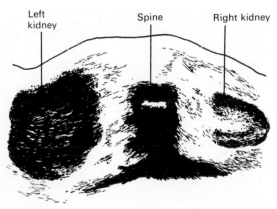

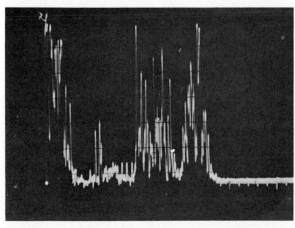

B

8.14 Renal masses—renal carcinoma invading the liver

Excretory urography indicated a mass in the right kidney of this middle-aged female. A longitudinal parasagittal section through the liver demonstrates that the only normal renal structure is in the lower pole of the right kidney. There is an ill-defined mass involving the remainder of the kidney which has internal echoes and attenuates the ultrasound beam. In addition, the only normal liver tissue is at its inferior aspect and anteriorly beneath the diaphragm. The remainder of the liver is replaced by tumor, as indicated by the lower level irregular echoes throughout. There is no demarcation between the upper portion of the kidney and the liver, a finding typical of direct invasion of the liver by a renal carcinoma. It is thus imperative that an optimal scan of the liver be obtained, as well as of the kidney, when evaluating renal mass lesions. Local invasion and blood-borne metastatic disease to the liver can then be readily recognized.

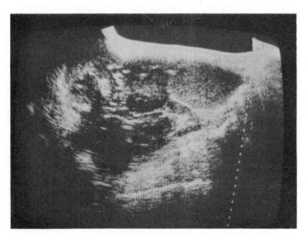
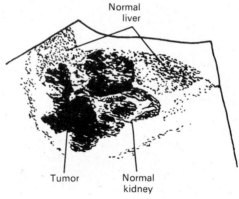

8.15 Renal masses—the anatomic splenic flexure as a renal imposter

The anatomic splenic flexure is that portion of the colon which is laterally placed below the tip of the spleen. The normal position of the flexure is considered reliable evidence that there is renal tissue in the left renal fossa (Moscatello and Lebowitz, 1976). The posterior portion of the left colon has been described as lying medial to the stomach in the left renal fossa in cases of renal agenesis or ectopia (Meyers, Whalen, Evans, and Viamonte, 1973; Moscatello and Lebowitz, 1976). In these cases, a pitfall in the ultrasound examination of patients exists. If the splenic flexure is fluid-filled, it may mimic a renal cyst or renal cystic disease. If, however, it is filled with feces, it may mimic a solid mass in the renal fossa (Teele, Rosenfield, and Freedman, 1977).

A. and B. This 15-year-old male was admitted with right flank pain. The excretory urogram demonstrates a hypertrophied right kidney and a medial splenic flexure (A). (The arrows indicate the direction in which barium would flow in a barium enema.) Bistable ultrasound examination of the renal area shows a normal right kidney and a mass with central echoes, suggesting a kidney in the left renal fossa (B). Identification of the anatomic splenic flexure placed medially in the region of the renal fossa on the urogram indicates that a left kidney is not present, and that the mass seen on ultrasound examination is the anatomic splenic flexure filled with feces. An additional clue on the transverse ultrasound scan is that the echoes which mimic the left collecting system are laterally placed.

C. A gray scale ultrasound examination of this patient done at a later date shows that the previously noted "kidney" has disappeared. There is no definite structure in the left renal fossa. A fluid-filled stomach is seen anterior to this region.

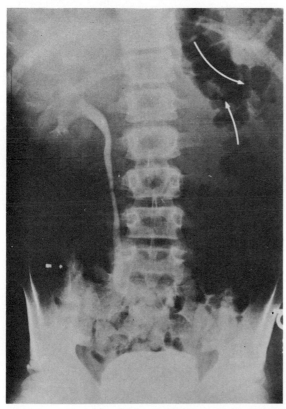

A

Left   Right

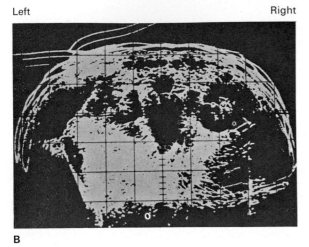

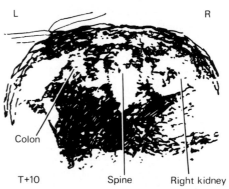

Colon

Spine   Right kidney

T+10

B

Left   Right

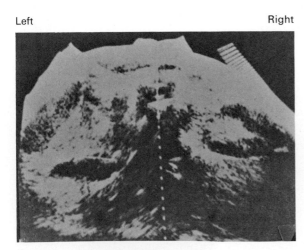

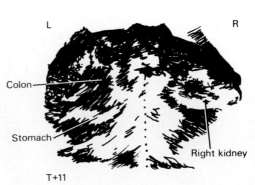

Colon

Stomach

Right kidney

T+11

C

8.16 Renal masses—ultrasound as a screening modality

Ultrasound is typically regarded as a method to evaluate known renal masses and is generally not used for initial screening. With the advent of better gray scale equipment, the renal parenchyma can be delineated and some masses identified which are not appreciated on excretory urography or nephrotomography.

A. For example, this is a representative tomographic section from the normal excretory urogram with nephrotomography of a 33-year-old male with hematuria.

B. Ultrasound demonstrates a mass in the lower pole of the right kidney which, although relatively homogeneous and not echogenic, does have irregular margins and significant attenuation leading to a shadow (s) behind it.

C. Angiography confirms the presence of a solid mass in the lower pole of the right kidney (arrowheads). At surgery this proved to be an adenocarcinoma of the kidney.

Ultrasound should routinely serve as a screening technique in patients in whom urography is not desirable due to a history of significant contrast media reaction, and in patients whose renal function does not permit adequate evaluation by excretory urography. In a patient with unexplained hematuria and normal uroradiologic studies, ultrasound is an additional, noninvasive modality to screen for the presence of renal mass lesions or other disease. Ultrasound provides an anatomic demonstration based on the acoustic properties of tissues and is independent of renal function. It is thus an invaluable complementary study to the standard imaging modalities.

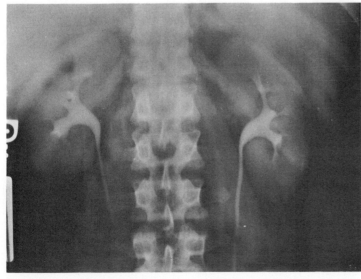

A

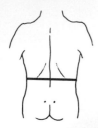

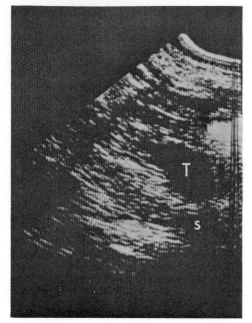

B

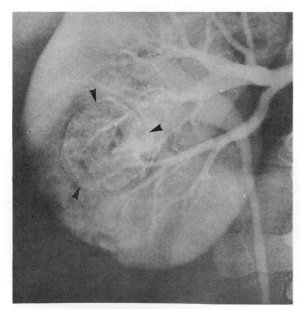

C

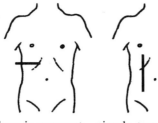

8.17 Hydronephrosis

A. Minimal hydronephrosis of the kidney is apparent as a slight separation of the normal central pelvocalyceal echoes. An intercostal sector scan (upper figure) is optimal to display the condition which is confirmed on longitudinal scanning (lower figure). This is a very sensitive indicator of urinary obstruction and minimal, transient distention of the collecting system may be produced by a full bladder.

B. With more significant hydronephrosis the calyces appear as dilated, fluid-filled structures, and the pelvis as a larger, fluid-filled structure. This is a simple transverse sector scan of the left kidney in a patient with moderate hydronephrosis. The dilated calyces can be seen leading into a dilated pelvis.

C. With more marked hydronephrosis the central collecting system may appear as a lobulated echo-free zone.

D. In severe hydronephrosis, the pelvis may appear as a large, fluid-filled zone in the kidney with the fingerlike projections representing the dilated calyces and infundibula.

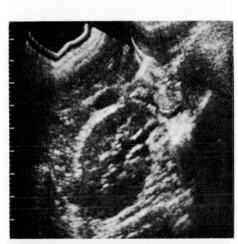

upper

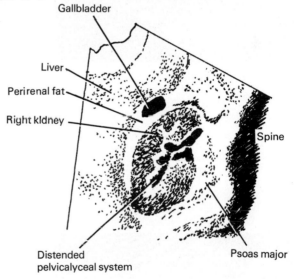

Gallbladder

Liver

Perirenal fat

Right kidney

Spine

Distended
pelvicalyceal system

Psoas major

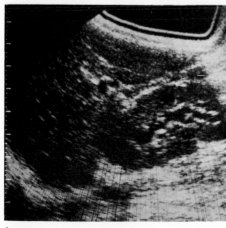

lower

A

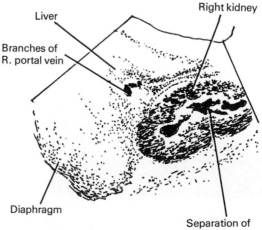

Liver

Right kidney

Branches of
R. portal vein

Diaphragm

Separation of
Pelvicalyceal system

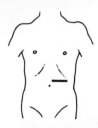

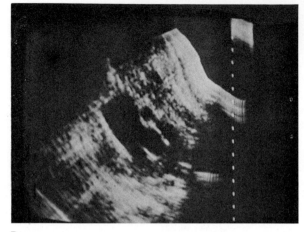

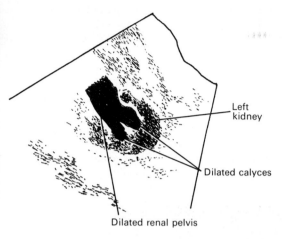

Left
kidney

Dilated calyces

Dilated renal pelvis

B

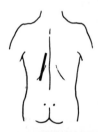

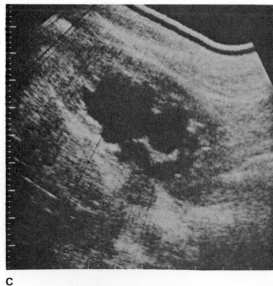

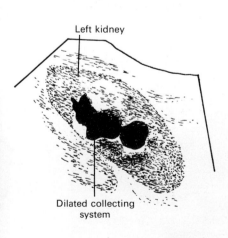

Left kidney

Dilated collecting
system

C

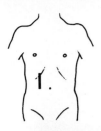

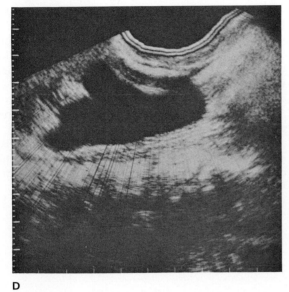

D

8.18 Hydronephrosis—congenital obstructions of the upper pole of the duplex system

A. This is a five-minute film from the excretory urogram on a 21-year-old female with stress incontinence. A mass effect is seen in the upper pole of the left kidney with inferior displacement of the visualized collecting system. There is also lateral displacement of the visualized ureter on the left.

B. A longitudinal section of the left kidney was obtained during the course of the urogram while awaiting delayed films. A normal lower pole central echo pattern is seen. The upper pole is an echo-free zone which is consistent with either hydronephrosis or a cystic mass. However, in addition, a dilated ureter is seen leading into the upper pole of the kidney. The most reliable way to distinguish hydronephrosis from a cyst,

whether there is a single or duplex system, is to identify the dilated ureter leading into the cystic structure. A dilated ureter cannot always be appreciated on ultrasound and, in addition, would not be present if the obstruction were at the uretero-pelvic junction or above this level. Thus the absence of a dilated ureter is not of diagnostic aid.

C. A delayed film at seven hours demonstrates contrast material in the dilated upper pole and ureter.

Surgery confirmed that this patient had a duplicated system with obstruction to the upper pole of the duplicated system. This ureter ended in the region of the uterus.

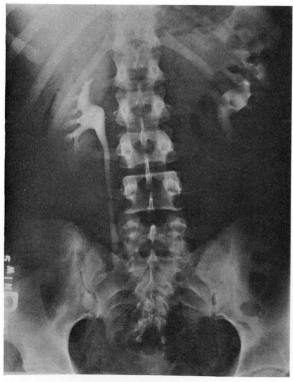

A

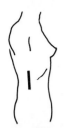

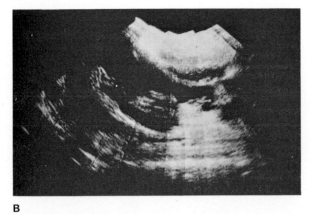

B

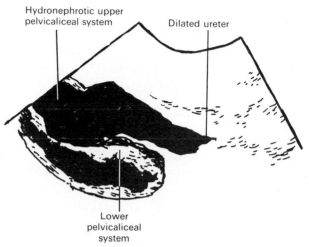

Hydronephrotic upper
pelvicaliceal system

Dilated ureter

Lower
pelvicaliceal
system

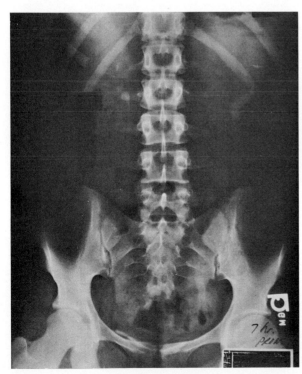

C

8.19 Hydronephrosis—Congenital ureterovesical junction obstruction

A.–C. This 6-year-old-boy presented with a large right kidney which did not function at excretory urography. A longitudinal parasagittal section through the right kidney with the patient supine (A) demonstrates multiple fluid-filled structures throughout the kidney. The transverse scan through the kidney demonstrates a similar pattern (B). Examination of the upper abdomen failed to reveal a dilated ureter, perhaps because of overlying bowel gas. However, ultrasound examination in the right true pelvis demonstrates a tortuous, fluid-filled structure consistent with a dilated ureter (C). At surgery this patient was found to have obstruction at the ureterovesical junction, presumably on a congenital basis.

If a dilated ureter is not appreciated when examining the region of the kidney, it is important to examine the true pelvis for evidence of a dilated ureter. Finding a dilated ureter permits the differentiation between renal cystic disease and obstructive uropathy. However, if a dilated ureter is not seen, one may not be able to distinguish between these two entities, particularly if there is ureteropelvic junction obstruction.

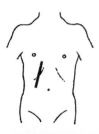

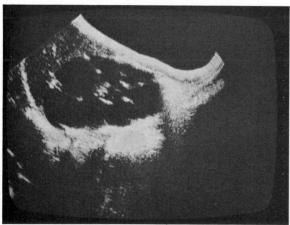

A

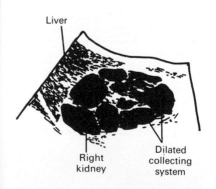

Liver

Right
kidney

Dilated
collecting
system

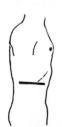

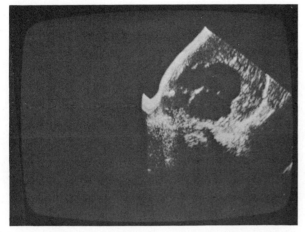

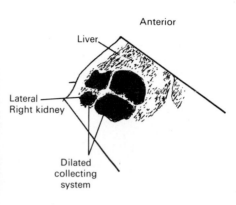

Anterior

Liver

Lateral
Right kidney

Dilated
collecting
system

B

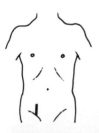

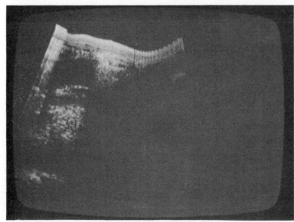

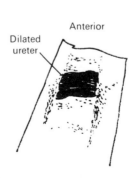

Anterior

Dilated
ureter

C

8.20 Hydronephrosis—staghorn calculus with hydronephrosis

A. This elderly woman had similar findings in both kidneys. In the right kidney, shown here, there is a fluid-filled structure occupying most of the kidney. In addition, in the medial aspect of the kidney there is a collection of high-level echoes with shadowing behind it. This combination of hydronephrosis and high-level echoes with shadowing is typical of a calculus obstruct-ing the renal pelvis. It should be noted that the presence of high-level echoes and shadowing associated with the calculus is not dependent upon the presence of calcium within the stone.

B. Excretory urography verifies the presence of bilateral staghorn calculi in this patient.

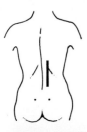

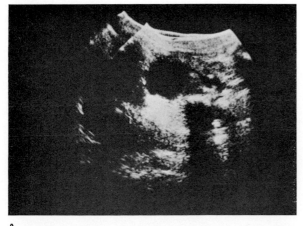

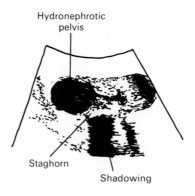

A

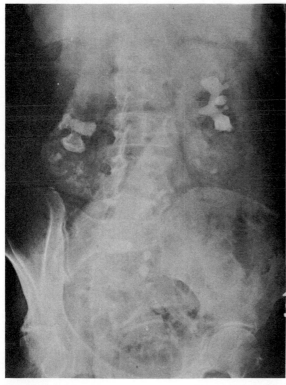

B

8.21 Hydronephrosis—pyonephrosis

This 22-year-old female presented with a history of recurrent right-sided pain of unknown etiology. An appendectomy was performed at another institution. Six weeks following the surgery, the patient developed fever and right upper quadrant abdominal pain. This was clinically felt to be a right upper quadrant abscess, and ultrasound examination was performed to further evaluate the patient.

A. and B. Both longitudinal (A) and transverse (B) sections through the right kidney demonstrate marked hydronephrosis. In addition to the hydronephrosis, however, ill-defined echoes were noted within the dilated collecting system, representing cellular debris—and most consistent with the diagnosis of pyonephrosis, presumably associated with an underlying long-standing obstructive uropathy.

C. Subsequent excretory urography confirms the gross hydronephrosis.

D. Retrograde examination demonstrates a partial obstruction of the uretero-pelvic junction.

At nephrectomy, the pyonephrosis and ureteropelvic junction obstruction were confirmed.

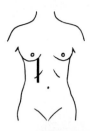

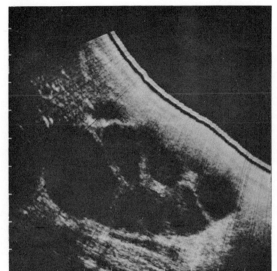

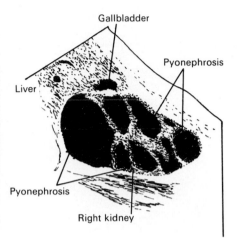

Gallbladder

Pyonephrosis

Liver

Pyonephrosis

Right kidney

A

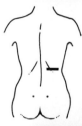

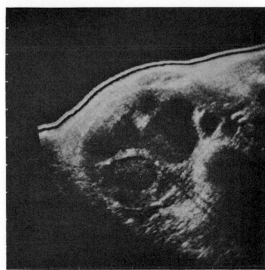

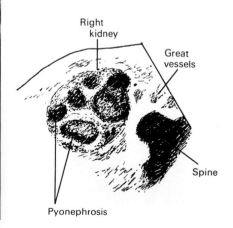

Right kidney

Great vessels

Spine

Pyonephrosis

B

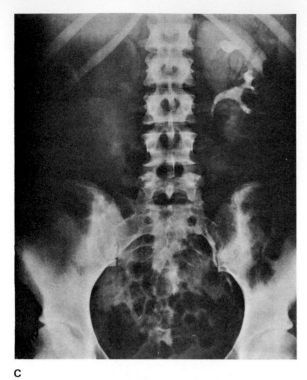

C

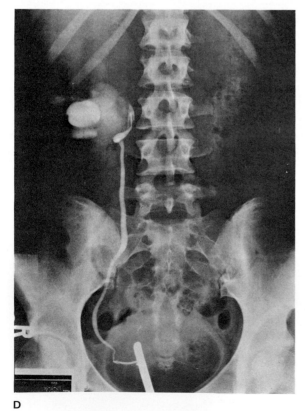

D

224

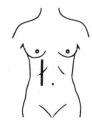

8.22 Hydronephrosis—of pregnancy

Hydronephrosis during pregnancy is a common finding, particularly during the later stages of pregnancy. There is a higher incidence of urinary tract infection during pregnancy as well. Excretory urography is not desirable for routine screening during pregnancy because of the irradiation to the fetus. Ultrasound examination of the urinary tract is a safe method of imaging which can diagnose anatomical abnormalities without using ionizing radiation. Hydronephrosis during pregnancy can be recognized by the separation of the normal central pelvicalyceal echoes. The kidneys may be more difficult to image in the pregnant woman, but the use of sector scanning will generally permit an adequate examination to be done.

This 24-year-old pregnant female presented with right upper quadrant pain. The clinical impression was that most likely there was urinary tract disease on the right. This longitudinal ultrasound scan through the right lobe of the liver and gravid uterus demonstrates the entire medical picture. The uterus is seen and there is a fundal placenta with the fetal head in vertex presentation. In addition, the mother's right kidney is well seen; there is separation of the central pelvicalyceal echoes, characteristic of hydronephrosis. The gallbladder is anterior to the right kidney. There are gallstones within the gallbladder, with the attenuation of beam behind the gallstones creating a "shadow" which obscures a portion of the kidney. The gallstones were felt to be responsible for the patient's symptomatology, and no radiologic procedures were required for further diagnosis.

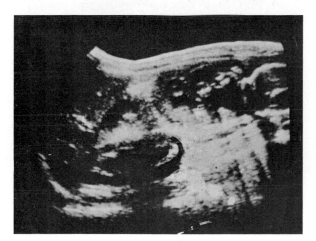

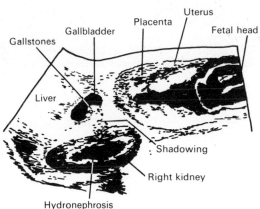

225

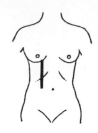

8.23 Renal cystic disease—adult polycystic kidney disease and liver disease

This middle-aged female presented initially in renal failure, which was subsequently diagnosed as adult polycystic disease. This longitudinal parasagittal section through the liver and right kidney demonstrates multiple echo-free zones of varying size throughout the right kidney, typical of cysts. The left kidney was similar in appearance. There are also multiple echo-free zones throughout the liver parenchyma, including one large zone in the posterior aspect of the right lobe of the liver. This pattern at ultrasonography is characteristic of adult polycystic kidney disease. However, approximately two-thirds of patients with adult polycystic kidney disease will not have hepatic cysts.

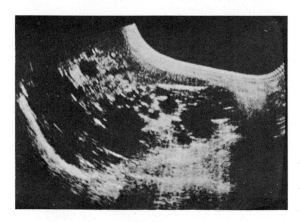

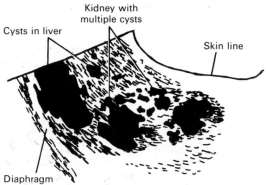

8.24 Renal cystic disease—multicystic renal dysplasia

The most common abdominal mass presenting during the first week of life is the multicystic dysplastic kidney, but this may be asymptomatic and present at any age. On ultrasound examination these lesions typically show a characteristic pattern consisting of a predominantly cystic mass containing septa which divide the mass into cysts varying in size (Bearman, Hine, and Saunders, 1976). On occasion this may present as a single large cyst.

A. This is a sagittal examination through the left kidney of a 15-day-old infant with a multicystic dysplastic kidney demonstrating a cystic structure (C) with several septa.

B. A longitudinal scan through the right kidney in a 7-day-old infant with a multicystic dysplastic kidney is shown. There are multiple cystic structures, and an arrow depicts the largest cyst present.

C. This figure demonstrates a cystic structure (C) with an irregular septum representing a multicystic dysplastic kidney in another patient.

D. The other pattern of multicystic dysplastic kidney in which one cyst predominates is shown, with a single large cyst (C) containing no internal echoes. This pattern cannot readily be distinguished from hydronephrosis secondary to ureteropelvic junction obstruction.

(Illustration reproduced by kind permission of Roger C. Saunders, B.M., M.R.C.P., F.F.R., Johns Hopkins University, Baltimore, Maryland.)

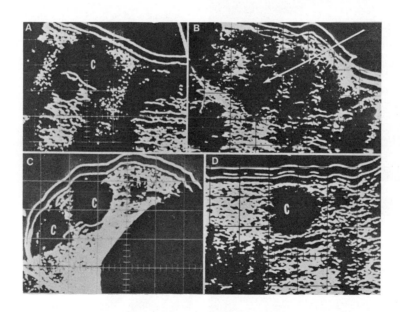

8.25 Renal carbuncle

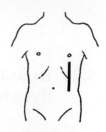

A. This 8-year-old male was admitted with a one week history of upper respiratory symptoms and a four day history of left-sided pain and fever. An IVP performed prior to admission had demonstrated a 7 cm mass in the lower pole of the left kidney. This longitudinal parasagittal section through the left kidney demonstrates a mass which is echogenic in the lower pole of the left kidney. Although these findings can be seen in either neoplastic disease or with a renal carbuncle, in view of the history a carbuncle was considered most likely. Renal arteriography was also consistent with this diagnosis. The patient was treated with antibiotics with regression of symptoms.

B. A longitudinal section through the left kidney performed five months after the initial study de-

monstrates a significant decrease in size of the previously described renal carbuncle. In addition, the lesion is now relatively echo-free. It is common for a carbuncle or abscess of the kidney to appear initially as a complex lesion containing echoes and subsequently under therapy to become echo-free. Thus, depending upon the time at which one sees the patient, a carbuncle may mimic a solid tumor of the kidney or a cyst. Appropriate history will generally permit the correct diagnosis to be made. Arteriography may be necessary to confirm the diagnosis, but surgery can generally be avoided. Percutaneous puncture of the carbuncle under ultrasound guidance may be useful both to identify the nature of the lesion and to culture the fluid.

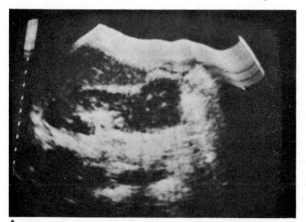

A

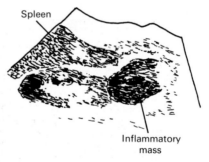

Spleen

Inflammatory mass

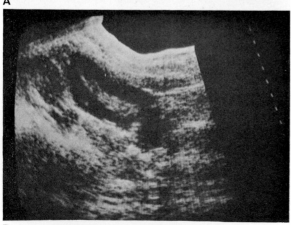

B

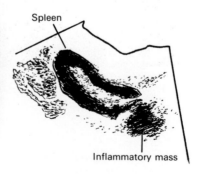

Spleen

Inflammatory mass

8.26 Inflammatory disease—perinephric abscess

Perinephric disease, such as abscess or hematoma, appears as a mass effect around the kidney. Typically these are relatively echo-free—although they may be echogenic, depending upon the amount of debris or organization within them.

A. Excretory urography on a febrile 54-year-old man shows a nonfunctioning left kidney.

B. This transverse ultrasound section with the patient prone demonstrates the tip of the right kidney and shows that beyond the posterior margin of the left kidney

(arrowheads) is a crescent-shaped, relatively echo-free collection, labeled A. This finding is characteristic of a perinephric collection.

C. A longitudinal section through the left kidney demonstrates that this collection extends inferiorly from this kidney, a finding typical of perinephric collections (Meyers, Whalen, Peele et al., 1972).

Since the patient had a history of fever, the correct diagnosis of perirenal abscess could be made from the ultrasound examination.

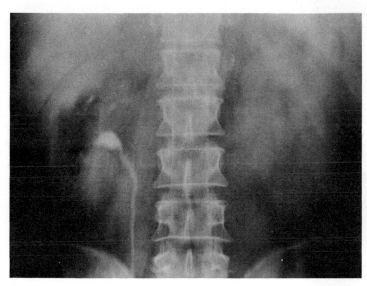

A

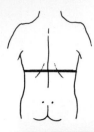

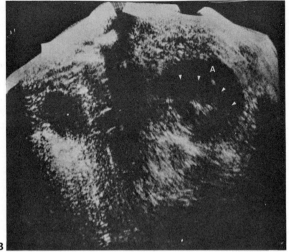

B

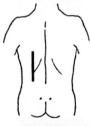

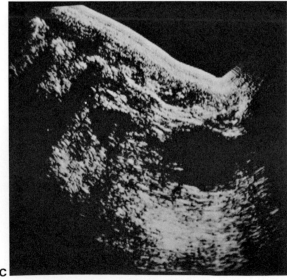

C

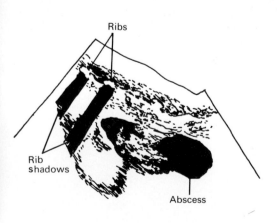

Ribs

Rib shadows

Abscess

230

8.27 Abscess in the true pelvis

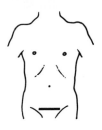

A 5-week-old boy was admitted with rising BUN after being treated at another hospital for dehydration and diarrhea. On admission, the WBC count was 25 000, and the patient was started on intravenous penicillin. Five days after admission, the patient's urine output dropped and he became edematous and hypothermic. An apneic episode was also noted. The right saphenous vein cutdown site exuded pus. A ^{67}Gallium scan showed diffuse uptake in the abdomen. Intravenous urography showed deviation of the bladder to the left. Transverse ultrasound scans of the pelvis reveal a homogeneous mass filling the right side of the pelvis and encroaching on the lumen of the bladder, one of which is shown here. The appearance is consistent with an inflammatory or neoplastic mass. Surgery was performed and approximately 80 cc of purulent material were drained from a pelvic abscess. Follow-up examinations and appropriate antibiotic therapy showed the mass to decrease in size.

This abscess was not localized by a Gallium study, which is unusual. In our experience, nonspecific uptake of ^{67}Gallium by tumor, abscess, wounds, and in the gut are more common problems. Because of these difficulties, we have found ultrasound a useful modality in the diagnosis of abdominal and pelvic abscesses (see p. 78).

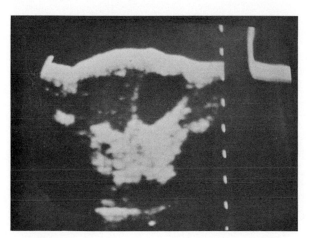

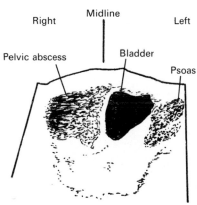

8.28 Miscellaneous—infarction

Infarction of renal parenchyma leads to deposition of collagen. The echo formation from collagen leads to high-level echoes in the zone of the infarction.

A. This middle-aged woman with mitral stenosis and atrial fibrillation has scarring of the kidneys, with normal collecting systems shown on excretory urography.

B. The longitudinal parasagittal ultrasound examination of the right kidney demonstrates loss of parenchyma; but, in addition, there are increased echoes within the parenchyma at the region of scarring—presumably corresponding to the region of deposition of collagen.

The finding of the normal calyces on the urogram and the scarring with increased echoes on the ultrasound study is a pattern typical of renal infarction.

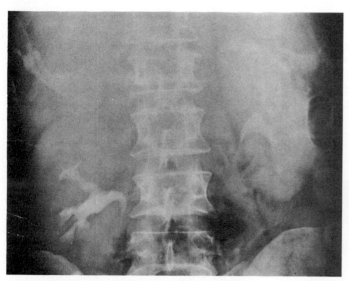

A

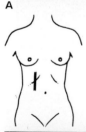

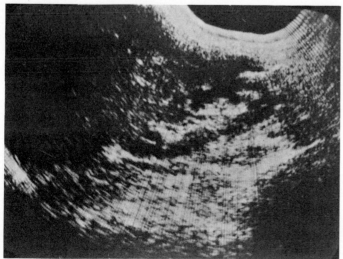

B

233

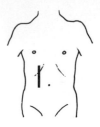

8.29 Miscellaneous—diabetic glomerulosclerosis

This is a longitudinal parasagittal section through the liver and right kidney of a 62-year-old patient in renal failure secondary to diabetic glomerulosclerosis. The left kidney was similar to the right. High-level echoes are seen emanating from the central pelvocalyceal system. In addition, the cortex is extremely well defined with higher than normal level echoes seen for the gain setting used. Because the cortex is so echogenic, the medullary region is well defined. The renal pyramids, particularly those seen adjacent to the liver, appear as echo-free zones. In diabetic glomerulosclerosis (Kimmelstiel–Wilson disease) there is an increase in mesangial matrix and in collagen. Other diseases which result in the deposition of collagen within the cortex, such as chronic glomerulonephritis, would be expected to lead to a similar picture.

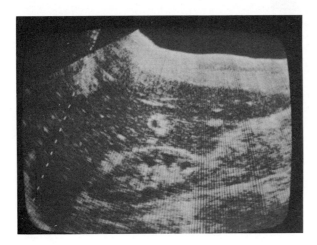

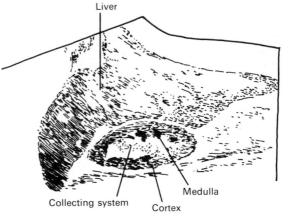

Liver

Collecting system   Cortex   Medulla

8.30 Miscellaneous—clarification of the excretory urographic study

Ultrasound is often a complementary modality in the clarification of an excretory urogram. For example, this 50-year-old female presented in renal failure.

A. Excretory urography demonstrates poor function of the kidneys. A pelvic density is noted, raising the question of a pelvic mass, enlarged bladder, or ascites.

B. A cystogram done at the time of urography demonstrates that the pelvic density is not the bladder.

C. Transverse ultrasound examination of the true pelvis demonstrates significant ascites, which shifted with change in position. The uterus is seen in the midportion of the ascites, with the broad ligaments well delineated.

D. Longitudinal ultrasound examination of the true pelvis once again demonstrates the uterus within the ascites. Therefore, the pelvic density which is seen on the urogram is definitely ascites. However, there is a "pelvic mass;" protruding from the superior aspect of the uterus is a solid, 1 cm mass almost certainly representing a small fibroid.

In addition, the ultrasound study demonstrated no evidence of hydronephrosis, eliminating obstructive uropathy as the cause of the patient's renal failure.

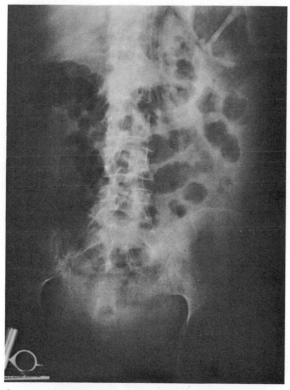

A

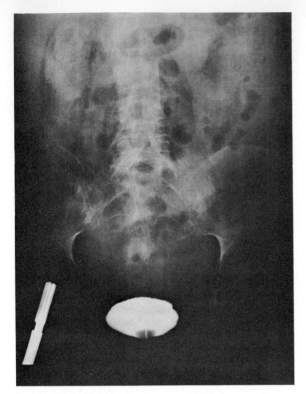

B

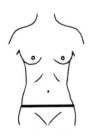

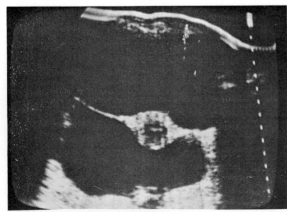

C

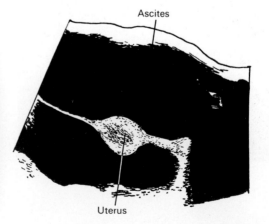

Ascites

Uterus

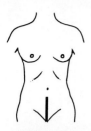

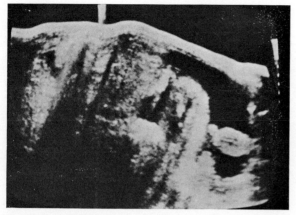

D

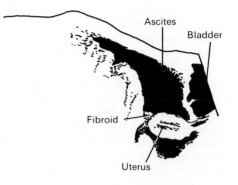

8.31 Renal transplant—obstructive uropathy

This 7-year-old boy received a renal transplant for renal failure due to long-standing obstructive uropathy. Postoperatively the patient was noted to have decreased urine output. Radionuclide evaluation was performed four days postoperatively, which showed normal profusion but delayed excretion, as well as a dilated pelvocalyceal system. Since an adult kidney had been transplanted, it was possible that the large renal pelvis might reflect the discrepancy in size between the transplanted kidney and the small patient. Ultrasound was therefore performed on the fifth postoperative day to clarify the radionuclide findings.

A. In this figure, the collecting system of the transplanted kidney is grossly dilated, a finding consistent with obstruction, but no dilated ureter is appreciated and no extrarenal fluid collection is visible.

B. Subsequent excretory urography confirms the presence of obstruction to the urinary tract.

C. A repeat ultrasound examination on the tenth day demonstrates continued dilatation of the urinary system.

D. It was elected to follow the patient. Repeat ultrasonography, performed on the 19th hospital day, shows a marked decrease in the pyelocaliectasis.

This case demonstrates the value of ultrasonography in initially diagnosing obstructive uropathy in the transplanted kidney at a time when such a diagnosis may be more difficult to make using excretory urography or radioisotope studies, since both require adequate renal perfusion and function. In addition, ultrasound provides a means of following these patients serially without exposing them to additional ionizing radiation or discomfort. As shown in Figure 8.33, when a mass lesion is present, such as a lymphocele or urinoma, it can be identified. Thus ultrasound has a potential to identify the nature of the obstruction or, equally significantly, to rule out an extrinsic mass as the cause of the obstructive uropathy.

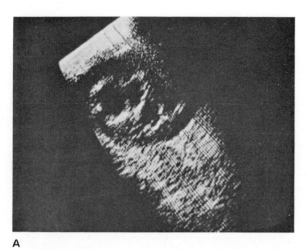

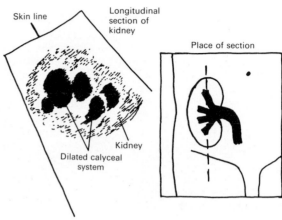

Skin line

Longitudinal section of kidney

Place of section

Dilated calyceal system

Kidney

A

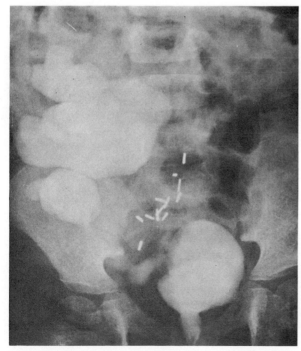

B

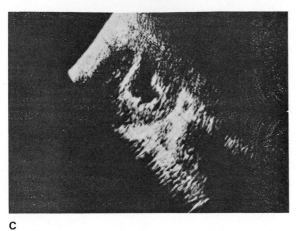

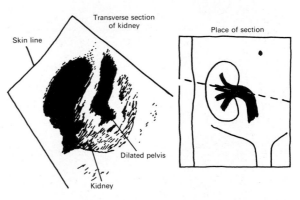

Transverse section of kidney

Skin line

Dilated pelvis

Kidney

Place of section

C

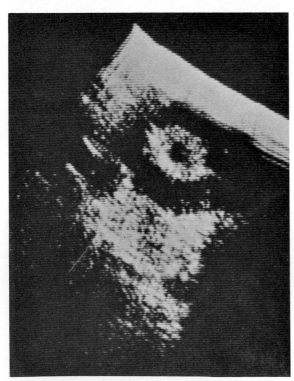

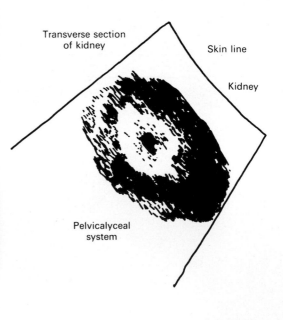

Transverse section of kidney

Skin line

Kidney

Pelvicalyceal system

D

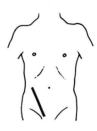

8.32 Renal transplant—rejection

This 16-year-old male had a renal transplant one year prior to admission and presented with a rising BUN and creatinine. Echo examination of the true pelvis demonstrated the transplant kidney. No pelvic fluid collection such as a lymphocele, urinoma, or hematoma was present. In addition, the central pelvocalyceal echoes were well delineated and there was no evidence of separation, as would be seen with hydronephrosis. An increase in renal size has been described with rejection and, therefore, if a previous ultrasound examination of the kidney is available for comparison one can accurately evaluate this parameter (Bartrum, Smith, D'Orsi, Tilney, and Dantono, 1976). In this patient one can appreciate the cortex as well demarcated from the medullary region. The intensity of echoes in the cortex is comparable to that in the central pelvocalyceal region. It has previously been suggested that high-level echoes may occur in the renal parenchyma with rejection (Leopold, 1970). In addition, the pelvocalyceal system is relatively small in size, suggesting surrounding edema. The kidney was removed and was found to be rejecting. This case demonstrates the significant role that ultrasound can play in complementing nuclear medicine and urography when evaluating a patient for transplant rejection. Ultrasound gives an accurate anatomic picture of the transplant and surrounding region, even if renal blood flow or renal function is poor, thus permitting obstructive uropathy and pelvic masses to be excluded.

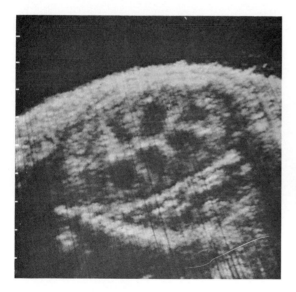

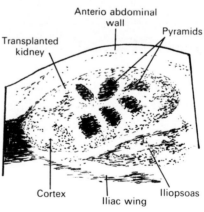

8.33 Renal transplant—lymphocele

Following renal transplantation, fluid collections such as abscesses, lymphoceles, urinomas, and hematomas may occur. Most of the time, these fluid collections are indistinguishable from each other and appear as sonolucent zones in the true pelvis. This oblique section of a renal transplant shows the transplanted kidney (TK) with a fluid collection (L) between kidney and bladder (B). This was aspirated under ultrasound guidance and proved to be a lymphocele.

(Illustration reproduced by kind permission of Roger C. Saunders, B.M., M.R.C.P., F.F.R., Johns Hopkins University, Baltimore, Maryland.)

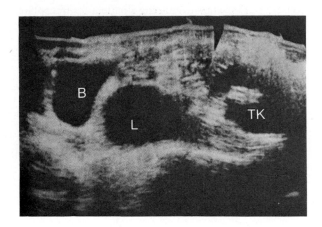

8.34 Adrenal pheochromocytoma

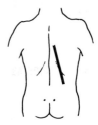

A. This longitudinal section through the right kidney with the patient prone demonstrates a mass related to the supermedial portion of the right kidney. This mass has a few low-level echoes within it, but is well defined and is approximately 3 cm in length.

B. Angiography verifies that a mass is present in the right suprarenal area and demonstrates that it is vascular.

At surgery a pheochromocytoma was removed. The adrenal regions are generally accessible to ultrasound examination. The right adrenal can frequently be seen with the patient supine, using the liver as a "window." In other situations additional projections, including the decubitus and prone positions, may be of aid in visualizing this area. Simple sector scanning through the ribs is also of use. Adrenal masses can be both identified and evaluated as to whether they are cystic or solid.

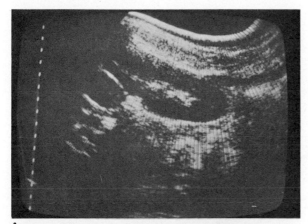

A

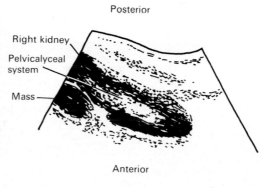

Posterior

Right kidney

Pelvicalyceal system

Mass

Anterior

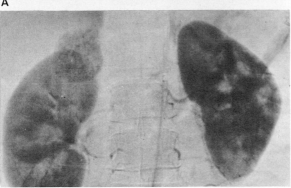

B

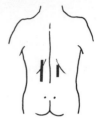

8.35 Adrenal—neuroblastoma

A. This 4-month-old child presented with a palpable left upper quadrant mass. This longitudinal ultrasound section through the kidney with the patient prone demonstrates a 6 cm mass above the left kidney displacing it inferiorly. The mass has irregular high-level echoes within it suggestive of calcification; it is clearly solid in nature. Excretory urography also demonstrated a mass above the left kidney with apparent calcification within it. In a child, any solid lesion found in the suprarenal area must be considered a neuroblastoma until proven otherwise. This patient had subsequent surgery which demonstrated the mass to be a neuroblastoma of the left adrenal.

B. This longitudinal section through the patient's right kidney with the child prone demonstrates a normal right kidney. Notice the punctate echoes at the cortico-medullary junction representing the arcuate vessels. The patient also had an ultrasound examination of the retroperitoneal area and of the liver, both of which were normal in appearance. In a child with a suprarenal mass, ultrasound can be of value in characterizing the cystic or solid nature of the lesion. In addition, should the mass be solid, areas of common metastases such as the retroperitoneal lymph nodes and liver can be examined for abnormalities.

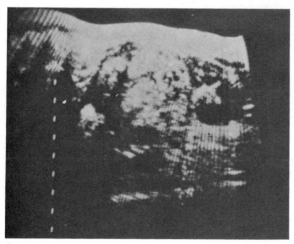

A

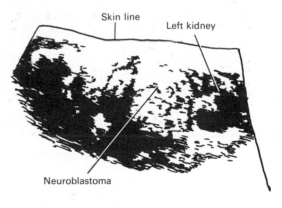

Skin line

Left kidney

Neuroblastoma

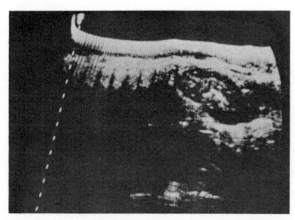

B

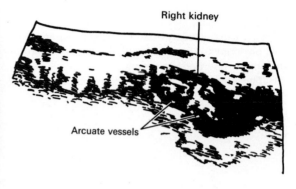

Right kidney

Arcuate vessels

8.36 Normal bladder—female

A. This is a transverse ultrasonogram of the bladder immediately above the symphysis pubis. The female bladder is rectangular on cross section. The fluid contents are indicated by a flat A-scan and inappropriate TGC posterior to the bladder. This excessive amplification partly obscures the uterus.

B. The uterus is displayed clearly on longitudinal section and can be traced inferiorly into the cervix and vagina. Low-level echoes may be seen in the bladder if there is debris present, or as an artifact in the obese. When attempting to assess whether an A-scan indicates a cyst or not elsewhere in the body, the bladder contents are useful as an internal calibrator.

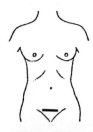

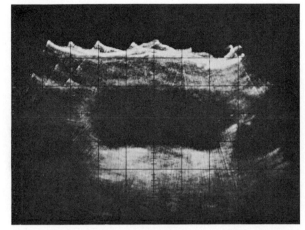

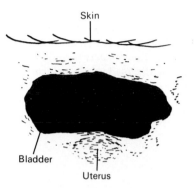

Skin

Bladder

Uterus

Transverse section
of bladder

A

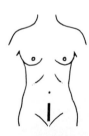

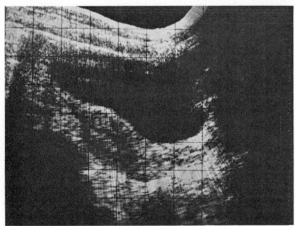

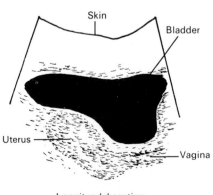

Skin

Bladder

Uterus

Vagina

Longitundal section
of bladder

B

8.37 Normal prostate and male bladder

A. This longitudinal section of the pelvis demonstrates a physiologically distended bladder. There are a few scattered echoes related to the anterior wall of the bladder secondary to reverberation. The prostate is well defined in the posterior aspect of the bladder. It has smooth margins.

B. A transverse section through the bladder and prostate demonstrates the prostate to better advantage. Note the high-level echoes delineating the outer aspect of the prostate and corresponding to the capsule of the prostate and its inner, less echogenic portion. The bladder lies anterior to the prostate.

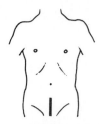

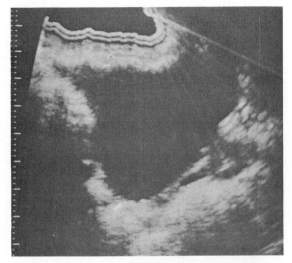

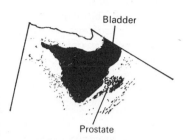

Bladder

Prostate

A

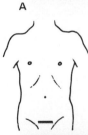

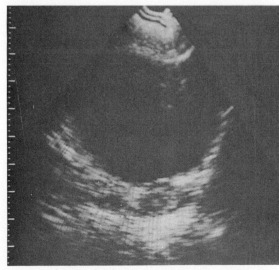

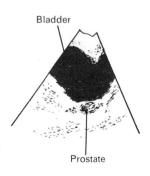

Bladder

Prostate

B

249

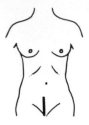

8.38 Bladder—carcinoma

A 66-year-old female presented with hematuria. Clinical examination and cystoscopy confirmed the presence of an advanced bladder carcinoma. A transverse ultrasonogram just above the symphysis pubis shows a sessile tumor arising from the bladder wall. The bladder wall is indurated and has lost its distended contour. There are also homogeneous strands of tumor material extending out towards the pelvic wall. These appearances have been described as indicative of malignancy in bladder tumors.

Bladder tumors frequently produce sufficient debris in the bladder to obscure the "clean" appearance of the wall. In this situation, bistable techniques are useful because such low echoes are lost. Alternately, the bladder can be washed out. This technique can be used to search for recurrence after surgical treatment of papillomata.

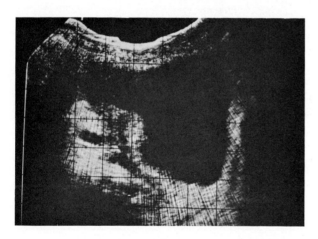

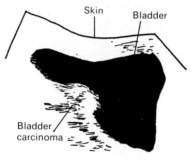

Skin   Bladder

Bladder
carcinoma

Transverse section
of bladder

8.39 Prostate carcinoma

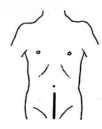

This longitudinal midline section through the bladder and prostate demonstrates the physiologically distended bladder. A rounded, fluid-filled Foley balloon is seen in the distal superior aspect of the bladder. Beneath the floating balloon is an enlarged prostate. The prostate is echo-containing but does not demonstrate good transmission. These findings are more consistent with prostatic carcinoma than with benign prostatic hypertrophy, which tends to demonstrate better transmission.

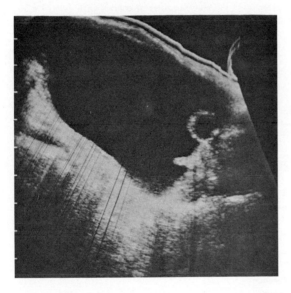

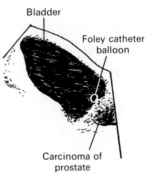

Bladder

Foley catheter balloon

Carcinoma of prostate

THE NONFUNCTIONING KIDNEY

The presence of a nonfunctioning kidney on excretory urography has become a major indication for renal ultrasonography. Table 8.4 lists the most common causes of a nonfunctioning kidney and ultrasonographic findings in each situation. Sections of this book that discuss each entity are also shown in the table.

clinician in determining what further studies are appropriate.

REFERENCES

Bartrum, R.S., Smith, E.H., D'Orsi, C.J., Tilney, N.L. and Dantono, J.: Evaluation of renal transplants with ultrasound. *Radiology*, **118**, 405–410, 1976.

Bearman, S.B., Hine, P.L. and Saunders, R.C.: Multicystic

Table 8.4 Nonfunctioning kidney(s) on excretory urography—ultrasonic evaluation

Etiology	Unilateral or bilateral	Renal ultrasound findings	Associated ultrasound findings	Figure(s)
Hydro-nephrosis	Either	Mild: Separation of the normal central echoes	Dilated ureter if the obstruction is beyond the ureteropelvic junction	8.17
		Severe: Echo-free central region, and/or multiple sonolucent zones	May see zone of echoes with shadowing with associated large staghorn calculus	8.20
			With pyonephrosis, may see echoes in the dilated collecting system from debris	8.21
Adult polycystic disease	Bilateral	Cysts in the kidney Nephromegaly	Hepatic cysts in $\frac{1}{3}$ of patients	8.23
Renal abscess	Usually unilateral	Mass in kidney. May be sonolucent or "complex."		8.25
Perinephric abscess	Usually unilateral	Sonolucent zone surrounding kidney which extends inferiorly		8.26
Renal infarction	Either	Renal size: Normal to small Renal parenchyma: Parenchymal echoes may be increased		8.28
Renal tumor	Usually unilateral	Echo-containing mass which attenuates the beam	Liver metastases may be identified	8.12 8.13 8.14
End stage renal disease	Bilateral	Small kidneys, normal appearance (may be increased cortical echoes with diabetic glomerulosclerosis or other cortical disease)		8.29
Renal agenesis or ectopia		No kidney identified in renal fossa	With left renal agenesis or ectopia, anatomic splenic flexure occupies left renal fossa	8.15
Renal vein thrombosis	Either	Nephromegaly may occur	None	
Multicystic dysplastic kidney	Usually unilateral	Fluid-filled areas with septation. Occasionally appears as a single fluid-filled sac.		8.24

In many situations—such as adult polycystic kidney disease, perinephric abscess, neoplasm, or obstructive uropathy—ultrasound may permit a definitive diagnosis. In other diseases, such as end-stage renal disease or renal vein thrombosis, specific findings are not seen at ultrasonography. Nonetheless, the ability to exclude certain disease states by ultrasonography will aid the

kidney: a sonographic pattern, *Radiology*, **118**, 685–688, 1976.

Cook, J.H., Rosenfield, A.T. and Taylor, K.J.W.: Ultrasonic demonstration of intrarenal anatomy. *Amer. J. Roentgen.* (in press).

Leopold, G.R.: Renal transplant size measured by reflected ultrasound. *Radiology*, **95**, 687–689, 1970.

Meyers, M.A., Whalen, J.P., Evans, J.A. and Viamonte, M.:

Malposition and displacement of the bowel in renal agenesis and ectopia: new observations. *Amer. J. Roentgen.*, **117**, 323, 1973.

Meyers, M.A., Whalen, J.P., Peele, K. *et al.*: Radiologic features of extraperitoneal effusions: an anatomic approach. *Radiology*, **104**, 249–257, 1972.

Moscatello, V. and Lebowitz, R.L.: Malposition of the colon in left renal agenesis and ectopia. *Radiology*, **120**, 371–376, 1976.

Raskin, M.M., Poole, D.O., Roen, S.A. and Viamonte, M.:

Percutaneous management of renal cysts: results of a 4-year study. *Radiology*, **115**, 551–553, 1975.

Rosenfield, A.T. and Taylor, K.J.W.: Grey scale nephrosonography: current status. *Journal of Urology*, **117**, 2, 1977.

Taylor, K.J.W. and Hill, C.R.: Technical notes: scanning techniques in grey-scale ultrasonography. *Brit. J. Radiol.* **48**, 918–920, 1974.

Teele, R.L., Rosenfield, A.T. and Freedman, G.S.: The anatomic splenic flexure: an ultrasonic renal impostor. *Amer. J. Roentgen.*, **128**, 115–120, 1977.

9. The great vessels

9.1 Aorta (longitudinal)

The abdominal aorta may be reliably identified on longitudinal and transverse ultrasound sections from the level of the diaphragm to the bifurcation at the level of the umbilicus. Initial attempts at scanning may show air-containing gut lying superficial to the great vessels, but repeated firm scanning movements in a linear plane should deflect any air-containing gut from the prevertebral region.

A longitudinal ultrasonogram 1 cm to the left of the midline (upper figure) shows the abdominal aorta in its longitudinal extent. The celiac trunk and the superior mesenteric arteries are seen; the latter is seen originating from the anterior aspect of the aorta at an acute angle. The superior mesenteric artery passes inferiorly into the root of the mesentery. The superior mesenteric artery separates the neck of the pancreas on its superficial surface from the uncinate process of the pancreas on its deep surface. The cephalic limit of the pancreas is formed by the celiac trunk and its branches.

A longitudinal ultrasonogram slightly to the left of the preceding section (lower figure) shows the superior mesenteric vein running parallel with the aorta and its bulbous termination as it meets the splenic vein to form the portal vein. In both these scans, the liver is seen anterior to the great vessels and has been used as an acoustic window to aid visualization of the prevertebral region.

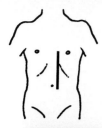

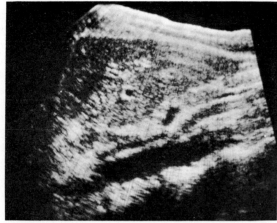

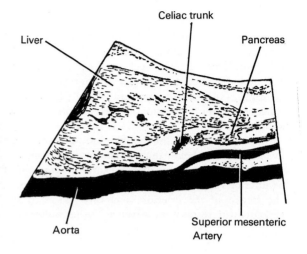

Celiac trunk

Liver

Pancreas

Aorta

Superior mesenteric
Artery

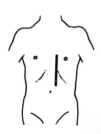

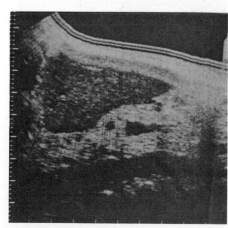

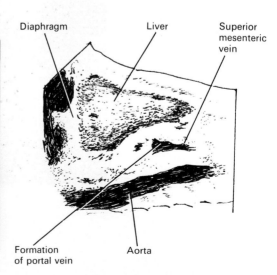

Diaphragm

Liver

Superior
mesenteric
vein

Formation
of portal vein

Aorta

255

9.2 Aorta (transverse)

The aorta is imaged by multiple sections at different distances below the xiphisternum. At the origin of the abdominal aorta at the level of the diaphragm the maximum diameter is 3 cm; this becomes smaller after the origin of the renal arteries and typically is only 2 cm in diameter at the bifurcation, which is at the level of the umbilicus.

Figure A shows the aorta and inferior vena cava immediately below the xiphisternum. The inferior vena cava is more anterior than the aorta, and the wall of the inferior vena cava is thinner than that of the aorta. The lumen of the inferior vena cava varies in size markedly with respiration as well as cardiac pulsations.

A transverse section 8 cm below the xiphisternum (Figure B) below the origin of the renal arteries shows a vessel of only 1.5 cm in diameter. The superior mesenteric artery is seen anterior to the aorta embedded in the fibrofatty tissue in the root of the mesentery, which appears as a highly reflective stroma around the superior mesenteric artery. The splenic vein is seen coursing around the prevertebral region and joins the superior mesenteric vein to form the portal vein.

A transverse section at the level of the umbilicus (Figure C) reveals the aorta in the midline with inferior vena cava more posteriorly placed.

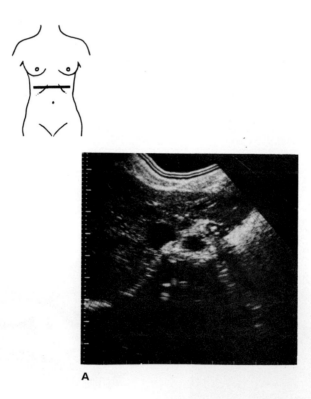

A

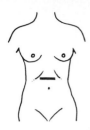

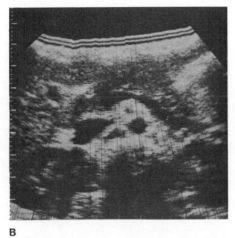

B

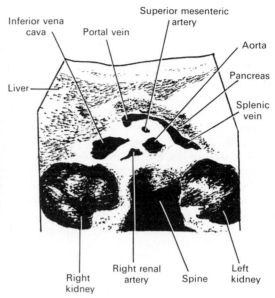

Inferior vena cava

Portal vein

Superior mesenteric artery

Aorta

Pancreas

Splenic vein

Liver

Right kidney

Right renal artery

Spine

Left kidney

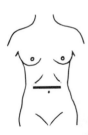

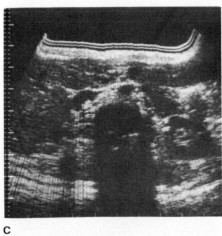

C

9.3 Branches of the aorta and portal vein

Longitudinal scan through the aorta may reveal the celiac trunk (see Fig. 1.9).

Transverse scans with the scanning arm directed cephalad show the celiac traunk and its branches (upper figure). Both the splenic artery and the hepatic artery are seen forming a "Y" with the main celiac trunk. The left gastric artery is not visualized. At this level, the right branch of the portal vein is seen lying anterior to the inferior vena cava. The portal vein and its branches have highly reflective walls which allow their differentiation from the hepatic systemic veins. The right branch of the portal vein is seen extending out into the liver substance, where it branches into anterior and posterior divisions.

The important anatomy is well shown on a limited section (lower figure). The hepatic artery is seen in immediate anterior relation to the portal vein, and it retains that relationship as both structures ascend in the free edge of the lesser omentum. Note that the splenic artery passes towards the left and becomes in posterior relation to the body of the pancreas. The precise identification of the lumen between the splenic artery and the aorta is not certain, but in some patients the fourth part of the duodenum (the duodenojejunal junction) is seen in this position and can give rise to confusing appearances both on ultrasound and CT scanning.

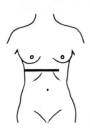

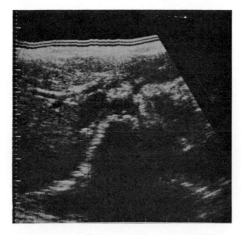

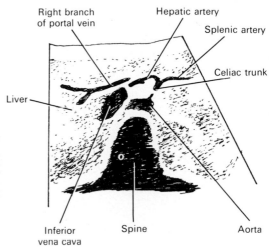

Right branch
of portal vein

Hepatic artery

Splenic artery

Celiac trunk

Liver

Inferior
vena cava

Spine

Aorta

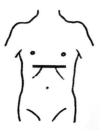

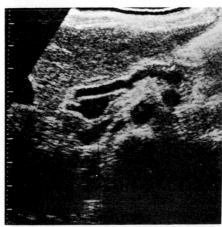

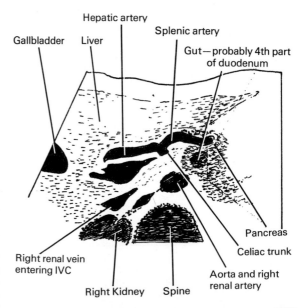

Gallbladder

Liver

Hepatic artery

Splenic artery

Gut—probably 4th part
of duodenum

Right renal vein
entering IVC

Right Kidney

Spine

Pancreas

Celiac trunk

Aorta and right
renal artery

259

9.4 Branches of the aorta—renal arteries

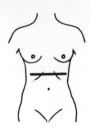

This transverse ultrasonogram shows the aorta with both left and right renal arteries. The inferior vena cava is seen receiving both left and right renal veins. The left renal vein is the only major vessel seen between the aorta and superior mesenteric artery. The medial end of the gallbladder is seen.

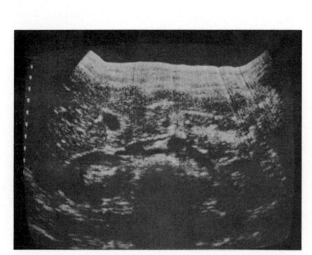

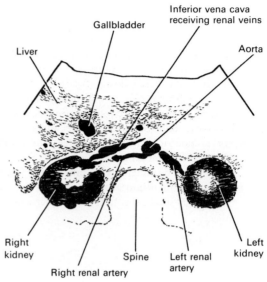

Liver

Gallbladder

Inferior vena cava
receiving renal veins

Aorta

Right
kidney

Right renal artery

Spine

Left renal
artery

Left
kidney

9.5 Aortic aneurysm

This 56-year-old male was referred for a palpable midabdominal mass. Ultrasound examination reveals a localized dilatation of the aorta, both on longitudinal (upper figure) and transverse (lower figure) sections. Note that the intraluminal clot is well demonstrated, which allows the ultrasonologist to measure both the lumen of the aorta and the size of the aneurysm. Arteriography is not only highly invasive but also provides only the former measurement.

Eighty percent of abdominal aneurysms involve the lower aorta and spare the origin of the renal arteries. It is, however, surgically important to try to predict when the renal arteries are involved. They can often be identified either by subxiphoid scanning, as in Figure 9.4, or by intercostal sector scanning, as in Figure 2.12.

The major advantage of ultrasound in the diagnosis of abdominal aneurysms is its lack of invasion, permitting repeated examinations over the course of months or even years. Aneurysms in excess of 5 cm require surgery, since they present an immediate danger to life. Smaller aneurysms may be treated conservatively since death from other manifestations of arterial disease is more common, and in such cases repeated ultrasound examinations form the basis of medical management.

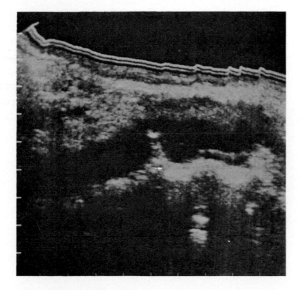

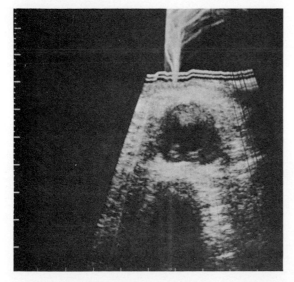

9.6 Aortic graft

This 60-year-old patient had an aortic aneurysm from the level of the renal arteries to the bifurcation of the abdominal aorta. At surgery, a Dacron graft replacement of the aneurysm was effected and the aneurysm shell sewn around it. A longitudinal ultrasonogram (upper figure) 2 cm to the left of the midline shows the entire extent of the abdominal aneurysm, the lower half of which has been replaced by the Dacron graft. There is a homogeneous material both anterior and posterior to the graft with some forward angulation of the graft. The transverse ultrasonogram (lower figure) 2 cm above the umbilicus shows the graft and the surrounding homogeneous area. These appearances simulate those of a dissecting aneurysm, but knowledge of the preceding surgery permits differentiation. The homogeneous area around the graft is clearly serous exudate and hematoma within the shell of the aneurysm. There is no evidence of leakage at the suture site, indicating that this is not a false aneurysm.

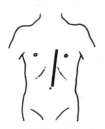

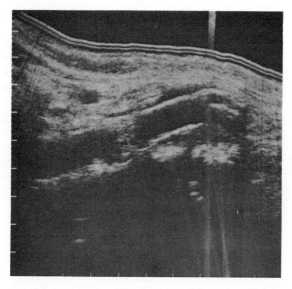

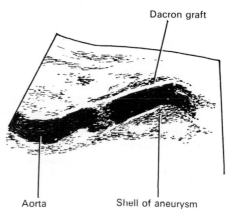

Dacron graft

Aorta

Shell of aneurysm

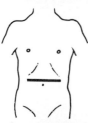

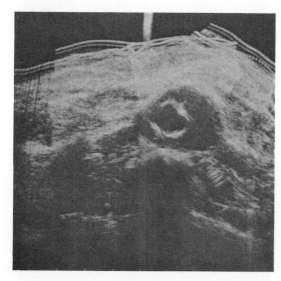

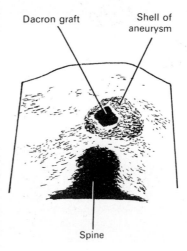

Dacron graft

Shell of aneurysm

Spine

9.7 Inferior vena cava and portal vein

This longitudinal ultrasonogram 2 cm to the right of the midline (Figure A) shows the inferior vena cava in its longitudinal extent. Unlike the aorta, the walls are thin and the vessel curves anteriorly as it passes through the central tendon of the diaphragm to empty into the right atrium. Since no valves are present in this part of the inferior vena cava or in its termination, the pulsations of the right atrium are transmitted down the inferior vena cava. The vessel therefore displays cardiac pulsations. In addition, there are variations with the respiratory cycle. In inspiration the increased abdominal pressure and decreased thoracic pressure ensure blood flow from the abdomen to the thorax, the respiratory pump. Thus a deep breath empties the inferior vena cava while a

prolonged valsalva maneuver distends the normal inferior vena cava.

These variations in the caliber of the inferior vena cava can be displayed using the M-mode (Figure B). The lumen of the inferior vena cava (L) shows large variations which are respiratory, whereas the smaller ones are cardiac in origin.

Figure C shows the origin and course of the portal vein. The bulb at the origin of the portal vein is due to the confluence of the superior mesenteric and splenic veins. From this origin, the portal vein ascends in a straight course in the free edge of the lesser omentum to the porta hepatis.

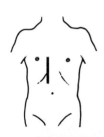

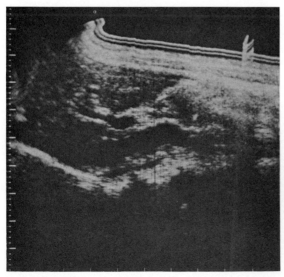

A

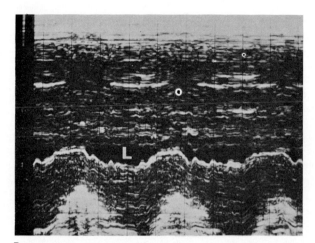

B

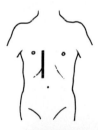

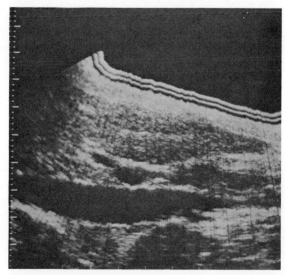

C

267

9.8 Inferior vena cava obstruction by malignant liver

This 55-year-old patient was known to suffer from chronic lymphatic leukemia and developed hepatomegaly and lymphedema of both legs. It seemed likely that there was pressure on the inferior vena cava. A paramedian ultrasonogram 2 cm to the right of the midline (upper figure) shows a grossly enlarged liver which is abnormally homogeneous, consistent with advanced malignant infiltration. The lumen of the inferior vena cava appears to be abnormally large below, while there is an apparent constriction at a higher level. An M-mode was taken below the level of the apparent obstruction in the plane shown by the dotted line.

The M-mode (lower figure) shows that there is no evidence for respiratory variations in the caliber of the inferior vena cava lumen (L), suggesting that the pressure changes in the thorax are not transmitted through the inferior vena cava and indicating obstruction to the cava.

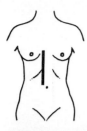

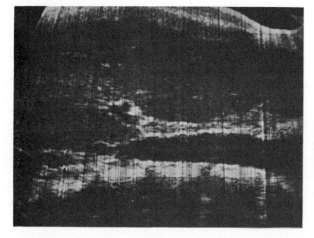

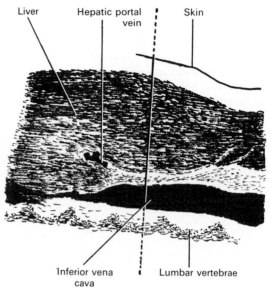

Liver   Hepatic portal   Skin
vein

Inferior vena   Lumbar vertebrae
cava

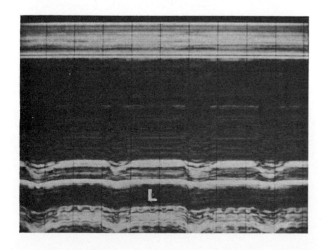

9.9 Inferior vena cava obstruction by para-aortic nodes

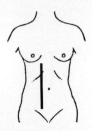

A 29-year-old farmer's wife had wide excision of a malignant melanoma two years before presentation with a large liver. Serology showed significant titres for brucellosis, and she was referred to differentiate between possible liver involvement by brucellosis and metastases from malignant melanoma. An ultrasonogram at that time showed homogeneous areas typical of malignant involvement. There was no evidence of the high-level echoes characteristic of inflammatory states (Fig. 4.48) throughout the liver and spleen. Serial scans were carried out on this patient during her terminal stages, when she developed bilateral leg edema. A paramedian ultrasonogram taken 2 cm to the right of the midline is shown. The liver is grossly enlarged and abnormally black. There is a lobulated mass in the para-aortic position, indicating lymphadenopathy. The lumen of the inferior vena cava is compressed by the lymph node mass.

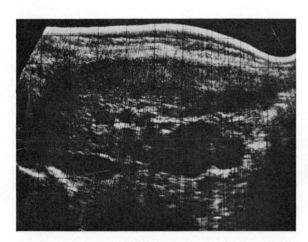

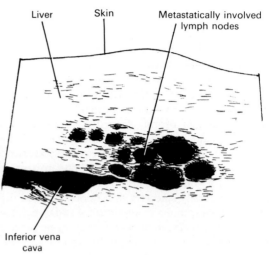

Liver   Skin   Metastatically involved
                 lymph nodes

Inferior vena
cava

271

OBSTETRIC ULTRASOUND SCANNING

Obstetrics is the most widely accepted application of diagnostic ultrasound because of the known hazards of ionizing radiation. The obstetric patient is requested to report for examination with a full bladder, since this produces an acoustic window to the pelvis by displacing air-containing loops of gut. A further advantage of a distended urinary bladder is that the cervix may be visualized and the relationship between the placenta and the internal os can be determined. The patient is scanned in the supine position. The surface of the abdomen is liberally smeared with mineral oil and the abdomen is then scanned in longitudinal and transverse planes. Longitudinal scans are taken at every centimeter from the left and right of the midline, and transverse scans are carried out at every centimeter above the level of the symphysis pubis. The technique involved in the determination of the biparietal diameter is detailed later.

INDICATIONS FOR ULTRASONIC SCANNING IN PREGNANCIES

There is an increasing argument that all pregnant patients should be scanned at least once during pregnancy to obtain an accurate maturity determination. The perinatal mortality in the United States is substantial compared with that of any other highly developed country. Postmaturity contributes to this high perinatal mortality. A single ultrasonic examination during pregnancy could exclude many other potential complications of pregnancy, including placenta previa, multiple gestation, and a gross congenital abnormality. While some of these conditions may be suspected on clinical grounds and thereby be referred for ultrasonic investigation, it is also possible for a patient to come to term without these abnormalities being clinically apparent. There is therefore a strong argument for scanning every patient at least once during pregnancy.

In a routine ultrasonic examination during pregnancy, an intrauterine pregnancy can be confirmed as early as four to five weeks after the last menstrual period. It must be recalled that the period of gestation conventionally quoted by obstetricians is dated from the last menstrual period, while fertilization occurs usually two weeks after this—so that an intrauterine pregnancy may be confirmed by ultrasonic examination at two to three weeks after fertilization or within a week of a missed period. Multiple gestation may be excluded at an early stage, since more than one gestational sac is seen in multiple pregnancies. A maturity estimation based on crown-rump length may be made between 6 and 12 weeks using the data published by Robinson (1973).

It has been widely reported in the literature using the older bistable machines that the biparietal diameter was not visualized until 13 to 14 weeks. Using the newer gray scale machines, a biparietal diameter is frequently identified as early as 9 to 10 weeks. However, the search for the fetal head at this stage is time-consuming; the easiest time to estimate fetal maturity by biparietal diameter is between 20 and 30 weeks of gestation. A routine ultrasonic examination during pregnancy includes localization of the placenta. During early pregnancy, the whole of the endometrium becomes thick and spongy to form an endometrial decidual reaction. With the implantation of the embryo, the future site of the placenta is determined. Ultrasonic scans of early gestation may show an apparent placenta extending around the whole wall of the uterus; the placental position should be determined later in pregnancy, when the position is better defined. In the third trimester of pregnancy, there may appear to be a substantial degree of placenta previa without the placenta completely covering the internal os, and these patients should have a further determination of placental position when they are nearer term.

There is a changing relation between the inferior edge of the placenta and the internal os as the cervix is taken up to form part of the lower segment. Thus a placenta which appears to show a major degree of placenta previa at 25 weeks shows no evidence of placenta previa at 35 weeks. This is sometimes referred to as migration of the placenta, but quite clearly there is no movement of the placenta relative to the wall of the uterus to which it is attached. There is merely differential growth, producing a changing relationship between the cervix and the placenta. This point must be remembered since there are two important sequelae. First of all, the migration of the placenta is always upwards so that a placenta which is fundal early will never become previa. Secondly, the changing relationship between the placenta and the internal os must be recalled when reporting placental position in the middle trimester or early third trimester. If any significant degree of placenta previa is seen, the patient should be rescanned at 34 to 35 weeks; in many instances it will be found that the placenta is no longer previa. If marginal degrees of placenta previa still persist at that stage, repeat examination at 37 to 38 weeks should be carried out. It is important not to risk an unnecessary cesarean section at 38 weeks based on the placental localization that was carried out at 30 weeks. However, if a central placenta previa is present, then any significant improvement is unlikely; but the placental position should still be checked immediately before cesarean section.

ULTRASONIC EXAMINATION OF ABNORMAL PREGNANCY

The most common problem arising in pregnancy is a uterus which is either too large or too small for the period of amenorrhea.

Uterus too large for dates

The most common cause for a uterus that is too large for dates is that the patient has got the date of her last menstrual period incorrect or that she has bled for one or two months while pregnant. Since the uterine cavity is not obliterated until approximately 12 weeks, the pregnant patient can bleed for the first three months of pregnancy. Other causes for the uterus being too large for dates include multiple gestation, polyhydramnios, hydatidiform mole, hydrocephaly, and a fibroid uterus. All these conditions may be separately differentiated, and examples are shown in this section.

Uterus too small for dates

Again the most common cause for a uterus that is too small for dates is an incorrect date of the last menstrual period. In early pregnancy, the possibility of missed abortion must be considered; this can frequently be discerned on the appearances of the B-scan, but attempts should be made to assess the activity of the fetal heart. With the ultrasound beam passed through the fetal thorax, the fetal heart can be seen to be pulsating. Alternatively, a Doppler device may be used and fetal circulation can be monitored. In later pregnancy, a uterus that is small for dates may be due to intrauterine growth retardation (IUGR). This is most commonly due to placental insufficiency. Comparison of the head and trunk size will assist in differentiating IUGR from the small fetus due to wrong dates. The starving fetus maintains brain growth at the cost of trunk growth so

that the head appears relatively large compared with the trunk. The trunk not only ceases to grow, but actually decreases in size as tissue is lost in starvation. IUGR can best be estimated by serial estimations of fetal size, both head and trunk.

Bleeding in early pregnancy

Bleeding in early pregnancy must be regarded as a threatened abortion, but other causes of vaginal bleeding should be excluded by clinical examination or ultrasonic investigation. The two important entities in the differential diagnosis which may be defined by ultrasonic examination are bleeding due to a hydatidiform mole and that due to a placenta previa.

Malpresentation

The presentation of the fetus can be very rapidly and accurately determined by ultrasonic examination. In malpresentation, such as a persistent breech presentation or transverse presentation, ultrasonic examination is important to exclude a possible cause for this—such as a placenta previa or congenital abnormality. A footling breech presentation is particularly important to recognize, since frequently it may be associated with prolapse of the cord and fetal distress; thus this must be recognized. At this medical center it is treated immediately by cesarean section.

Suspected fetal abnormality

If fetal abnormality is suspected, an ultrasonic investigation is an adequate method to exclude at least certain gross anomalies. Thus patients with a history of neural tube defects should be scanned early in pregnancy to exclude anencephaly. Careful examination of the spine allows a spina bifida to be recognized, and certainly a meningomyelocele. Similarly, in patients with polycystic disease, polycystic kidneys in the fetus can be excluded prenatally. In patients with suspected renal agenesis, the fetus can be scanned and the kidneys recognized. The fetal bladder can also be noted in a state of distention. The fetal bladder empties approximately every hour, and repeat scans of the fetus allow the urinary flow to be estimated. Normal urinary flow indicates normal renal function. Hydrocephaly can also be recognized, since the normal lateral ventricles can be seen on either side of the midline echo.

REFERENCE

Robinson, H.P.: Sonar measurement of fetal crown-rump length as means of assessing maturity in first trimester of pregnancy. *Brit. Med. J.*, **4**, 28–31, 1973.

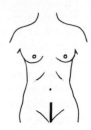

10.1 Normal development—5, 6, and 8 weeks' gestation

A. 5 weeks' gestation. This longitudinal ultrasonogram shows the gravid uterus lying posterior to the distended bladder. A decidual reaction is seen in the uterine cavity with thickening in the posterior wall to form the decidua basalis—the site of the placental formation. Fetal echoes are barely detected.

The position of the cervix may be estimated by the intersection of a line through the lumen of the vagina and a line through the longitudinal axis of the uterus. These lines meet at an angle approaching a right angle.

B. 6 weeks' gestation. This longitudinal ultrasonogram through the gravid uterus shows the decidual reaction in the uterine cavity and definite fetal echoes from within the gestational sac. The overall size of the uterus is larger than that seen in A.

C. 8 weeks' gestation. There has been further growth in the overall size of the uterus. The fetal heart can usually be detected by M-mode.

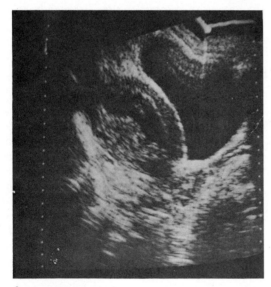

A

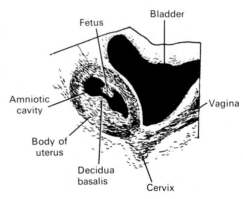

Fetus

Bladder

Amniotic cavity

Vagina

Body of uterus

Decidua basalis

Cervix

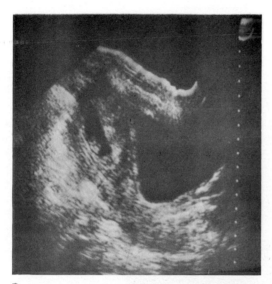

B

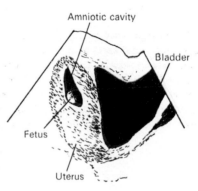

Amniotic cavity

Bladder

Fetus

Uterus

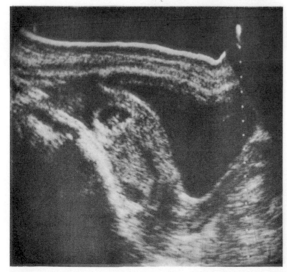

C

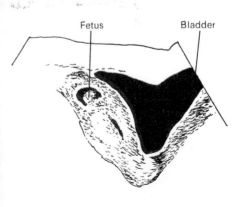

Fetus

Bladder

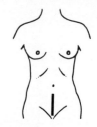

10.2 Normal anatomy—8 weeks' gestation

This 25-year-old female presented with a nine week history of amenorrhea, a mass in the left adnexal region, and a positive UCG. She was referred to exclude an ectopic gestation.

The transverse ultrasonogram seen in Figure A shows the gestational sac with the fetal parts within it, while a further section (magnified) shown in Figure B demonstrates the fetal head and trunk, which has a crown-rump measurement of 23 mm. When an A-scan was placed through the fetal thorax, fetal life was confirmed. Both atrioventricular valves are displayed on the M-mode recording in Figure C. These scans confirm that the pregnancy is intrauterine; there is no evidence of any ectopic gestation.

It used to be stated that the fetal head was not seen until 13 weeks; however, with the enhanced resolution possible with gray scale techniques, the fetal head is frequently seen before this, as in this patient in whom the fetal head was visualized at nine weeks. Of interest also is the demonstration of the fetal heart and the two normal atrioventricular valves at this stage of gestation.

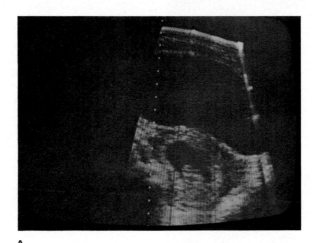

A

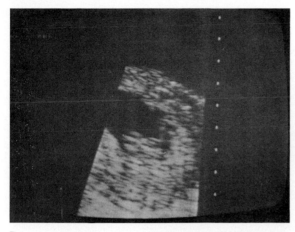

B

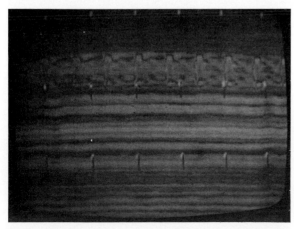

C

277

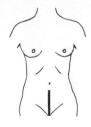

10.3 Normal development

A. 9 weeks' gestation. The overall size of the uterus has further increased and definite fetal structure is observed.

B. and C. 11½ weeks' gestation. The decidual reaction is seen around the entire uterus and there is fusion of the decidua parietalis and capsularis. The fetus is well seen on appropriate sections. The fetal head, trunk, and limbs are noted.

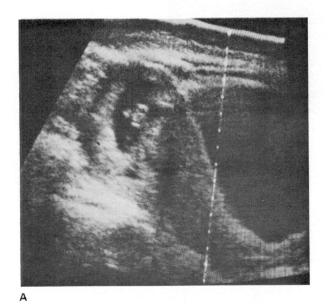

A

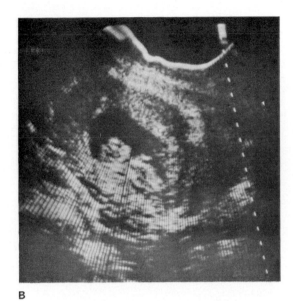

B

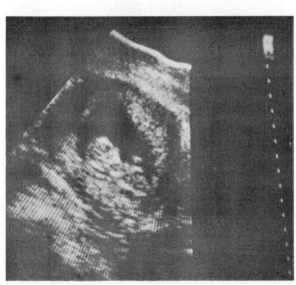

C

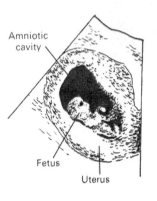

Amniotic
cavity

Fetus

Uterus

10.4 Normal development

A. 12 weeks' gestation. This longitudinal ultrasonogram through the gravid uterus shows a posterior placenta. The fetal trunk and limbs are seen free within the amniotic sac.

B. 16 weeks' gestation. An anterior placenta is seen. The fetus is well formed and is in breech presentation. The head, including the falx cerebri, is well displayed.

The vertebral column, ribs, and pelvic girdle can be discerned at this stage.

C. 21 weeks' gestation. A singleton fetus is shown in vertex presentation. An anterior placenta is seen. The maturity is estimated by the biparietal diameter seen on transverse scanning.

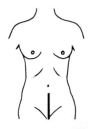

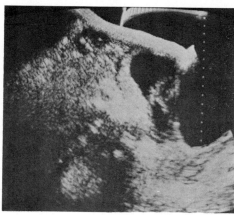

A

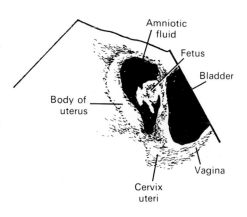

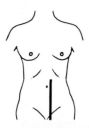

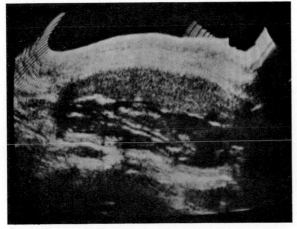

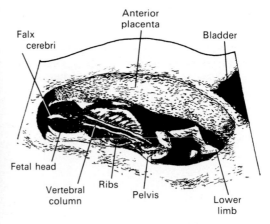

Anterior
placenta

Falx
cerebri

Bladder

Fetal head

Vertebral
column

Ribs

Pelvis

Lower
limb

B

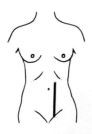

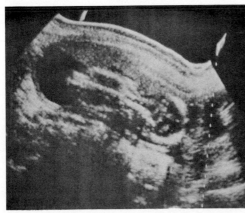

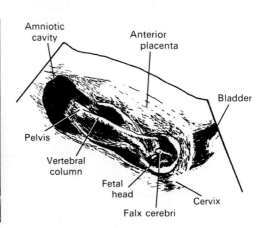

Amniotic
cavity

Anterior
placenta

Bladder

Pelvis

Vertebral
column

Fetal
head

Cervix

Falx cerebri

C

10.5 Normal development

A. 27 weeks' gestation. This longitudinal scan through the gravid uterus shows a singleton fetus in breech presentation with fundal and anterior placenta.

B. Transverse ultrasonogram of the same fetus as shown in A. The section is taken through the fetal trunk and shows the fetal arm. The anterior portion of the placenta is seen.

C. 28 weeks' gestation. A singleton fetus is seen in vertex presentation. The fetal legs are fully flexed at the hips and extended at the knees. An anterior and fundal placenta is seen.

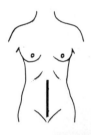

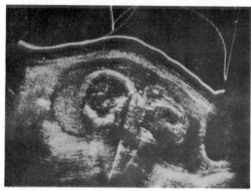

A

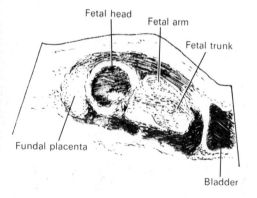

Fetal head

Fetal arm

Fetal trunk

Fundal placenta

Bladder

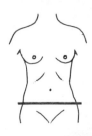

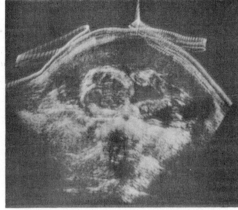

B

Placenta

Fetal arm

Spine

Thorax

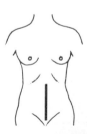

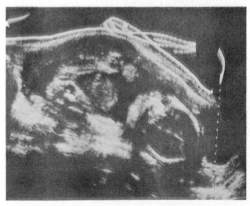

C

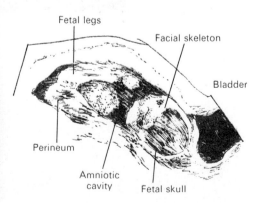

Fetal legs

Facial skeleton

Bladder

Perineum

Amniotic
cavity

Fetal skull

10.6 Normal development

A. 33 weeks' gestation. This longitudinal ultrasonogram shows a singleton fetus in vertex presentation. An anterior placenta is seen.

B. 34 weeks' gestation. A singleton fetus is seen in vertex presentation. Details of upper and lower limbs are displayed. An anterior placenta is seen.

C. 36 weeks' gestation. A singleton fetus is presented in vertex presentation. Transverse sections of all four limbs are seen. An anterior placenta is shown with early changes of consistency. More homogeneous areas are appearing, as well as flecks of high-level echoes, which are degenerative changes found in mature placentae.

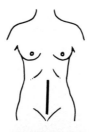

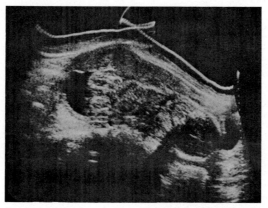

A

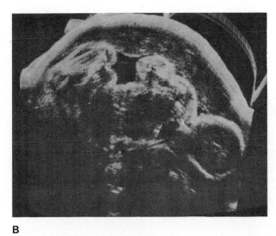

B

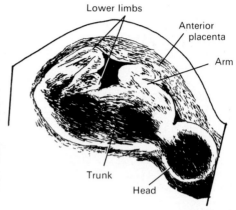

Lower limbs

Anterior placenta

Arm

Trunk

Head

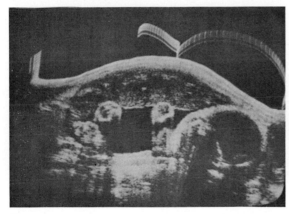

C

285

10.7 Placental maturity

The placenta is characteristically uniform in appearance up to about 36 weeks. Thereafter, an increasing number of placentae show heterogeneous changes with the characteristics of a mature placenta. The longitudinal ultrasonogram (upper figure) shows a fetus in breech presentation and an anterior placenta. The transverse ultrasonogram (lower figure) shows a section through the fetal trunk with a right anterior placenta. The placenta shows relatively echo-free areas, with high-level echoes around the circumference of these lobules. These high-level echoes may be associated with calcification within the placenta. Such changes are characteristic of aging and mature placentae.

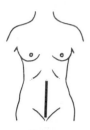

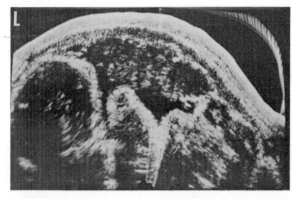

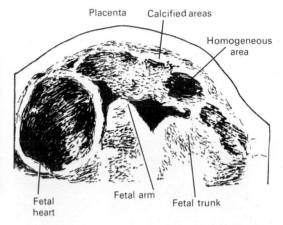

Placenta   Calcified areas

Homogeneous
area

Fetal
heart   Fetal arm   Fetal trunk

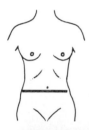

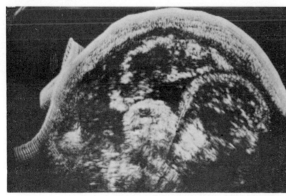

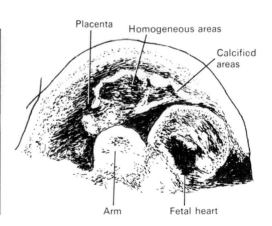

Placenta   Homogeneous areas

Calcified
areas

Arm   Fetal heart

10.8 Premature placental senescence

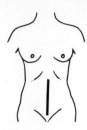

This patient presented at 34 weeks' gestation. Ultrasonic examination of the placenta reveals a chorionic plate, which shows an irregular edge. The body of the placenta shows homogeneous areas with high-level echoes, consistent with placental degeneration and calcification. Such appearances are frequently seen after 36 weeks but have poor prognostic significance when seen earlier in pregnancy. These changes of premature placental senescence are particularly noted in hypertensive patients.

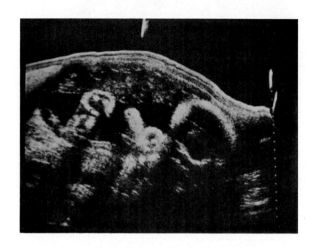

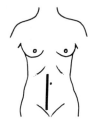

10.9 Normal anatomy—vertebrae, ribs, limbs

A. Single fetus is present in vertex presentation. The individual vertebrae and ribs are well demonstrated on this longitudinal section. The placenta is well seen posteriorly extending downwards from the fundus.

B. Single fetus in vertex presentation shows an anterior placenta. There is shadowing from the individual vertebrae, and a large fluid-filled gastric fundus can be seen.

C. Normal fetus of 18 weeks in vertex presentation. The lower limbs can be seen. There is a posterior placenta extending down from the fundus.

D. Normal fetus at term. The fetal head is in apposition with the placenta. The orbits and facial skeleton are clearly seen.

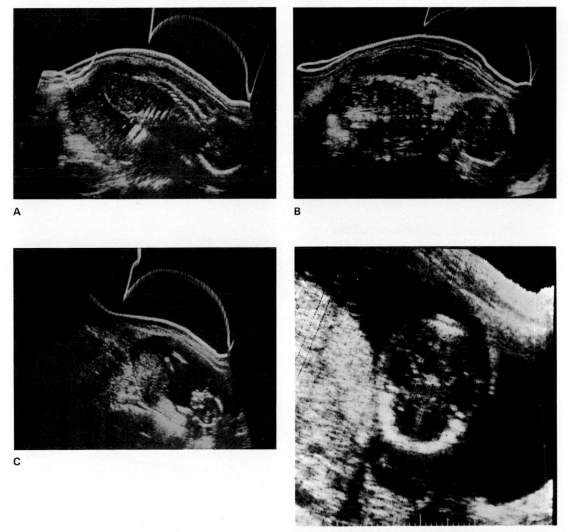

A

B

C

D

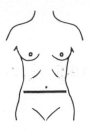

10.10 Normal fetal kidneys

The transverse ultrasonogram (upper figure) through the fetal trunk at 26 weeks' gestation shows both kidneys cut transversely with the spine between them. Fetal polycystic disease or renal agenesis can therefore be diagnosed. If renal agenesis is suspected the fetal bladder should be scanned, thereby demonstrating fetal urine production and hence functioning kidneys.

An oblique tomogram through the fetal trunk at 28 weeks (lower figure) demonstrates an oblique longitudinal cut through the kidney and a distended urinary bladder. Note that at least two pyramids can be seen (see page 191).

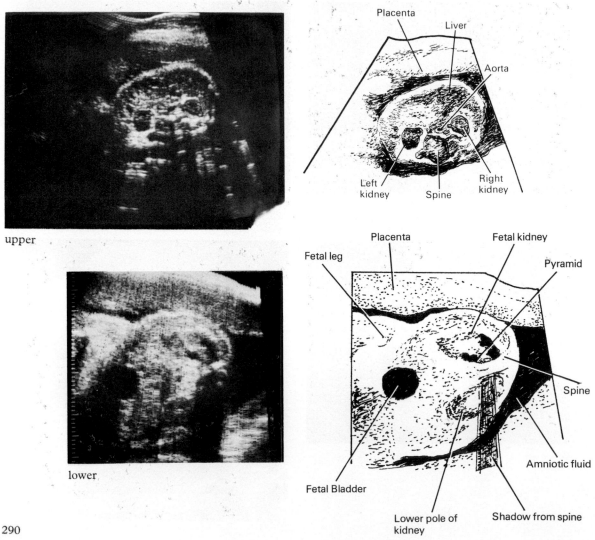

upper

lower

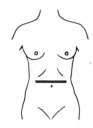

10.11 Normal anatomy—arms and fundus of stomach

This transverse ultrasonogram (upper figure) shows the fetal trunk and upper limb. The digits are seen. The placenta is seen anterior to the fetus.

The transverse section through the fetal abdomen (lower figure) shows the fetal liver and a distended, fluid-filled cavity within the left upper quadrant. This is the fundus of the stomach. This patient had polyhydramnios, which may be associated with esophageal atresia. This observation of fluid in the gastric fundus precludes esophageal atresia.

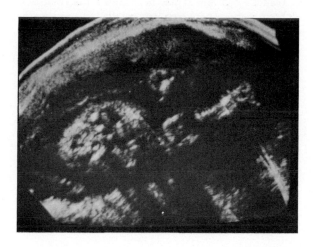

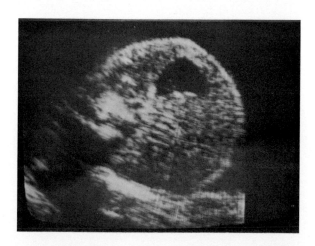

10.12 Normal anatomy—male fetus and bladder

A. Male genitalia are clearly seen in this transverse section through the perineum. At the present stage of the development of ultrasound technology, it is only possible to infer a female fetus by ultrasound examination after failure to visualize the external male genitalia. The frequency with which accurate sexing is achieved varies with the amount of time the ultrasonologist is prepared to spend making multiple sections through the pelvis. This is greatly facilitated by the use of a high-resolution real-time scanner.

B. This longitudinal ultrasonogram through the gravid uterus shows a singleton fetus in vertex presentation. The fetal liver is seen, pierced by the ductus venosus. In the fetal pelvis, a distended fetal bladder is well seen. The bladder can be observed to fill and empty approximately every hour. Estimates of the urinary volume flow can be attempted based on measurements of bladder volume. It has been noted that fetuses of diabetic mothers have high urinary flow, suggesting that they, like their mothers, have an osmotic diuresis.

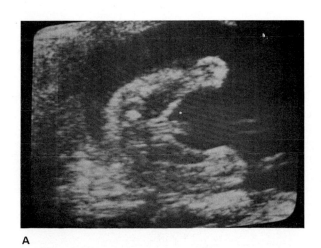

A

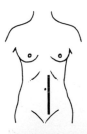

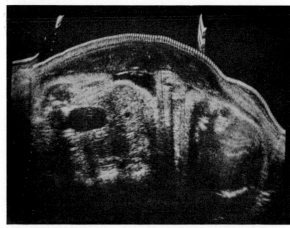

B

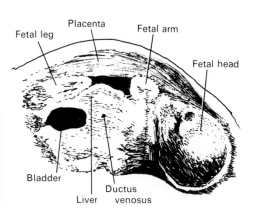

Fetal leg

Placenta

Fetal arm

Fetal head

Bladder

Liver

Ductus
venosus

10.13 Normal anatomy—umbilical cord and fundus of stomach

A. This transverse ultrasonogram through the gravid uterus shows a transverse section through the fetal trunk cutting the heart. Loops of the umbilical cord are clearly seen lying free in the amniotic fluid. An anterior placenta is well displayed.

B. Longitudinal ultrasonogram through the gravid uterus shows a singleton fetus in vertex presentation. The fetal heart is seen with shadowing from the fetal ribs. Below the diaphragm, the fetal liver is seen together with the fundus of the stomach. An anterior placenta is seen.

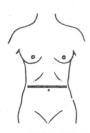

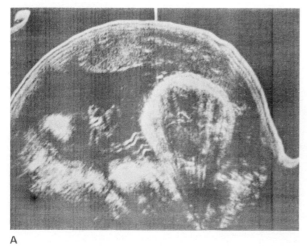

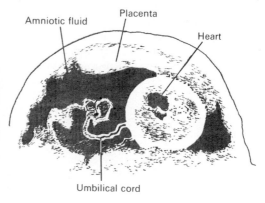

Amniotic fluid   Placenta

Heart

Umbilical cord

A

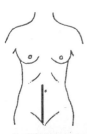

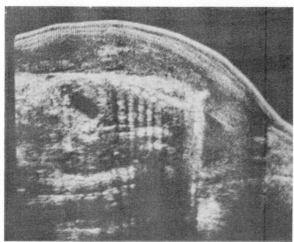

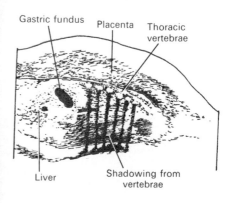

Gastric fundus   Placenta   Thoracic vertebrae

Liver   Shadowing from vertebrae

B

10.14 Normal anatomy—heart valves and M-mode

A singleton fetus is seen in vertex presentation. The heart has been recorded in diastole, resulting in unusually good resolution free of biological movement. Both ventricles are well seen, as is the aortic root. High resolution real-time machines which are currently becoming available enable the fetal heart to be displayed as it beats. However, the cardiac movements can be recorded using an M-mode tracing (p. 4). This is shown in the lower scan. Both ventricles are seen with recordings from both atrioventricular valves and the interventricular septum between them. Not only can fetal life be confirmed, but the technique can be used in a more quantitative way to monitor the fetal hemodynamics by measuring the preejection period (PEP).

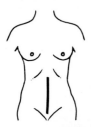

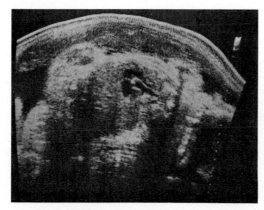

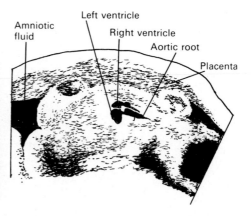

Amniotic fluid

Left ventricle

Right ventricle

Aortic root

Placenta

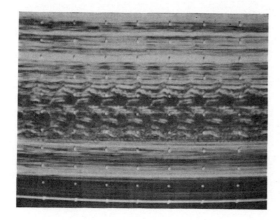

10.15 Fetal anatomy

A. A longitudinal scan of the fetus reveals the aorta throughout its length and the bifurcation of the aorta into the common iliac arteries. In the paravertebral region, the fetal kidney can be easily discerned (K).

B. This figure shows a transverse section through the fetal trunk in which the fundus of the stomach and the ductus venosus are seen passing through the liver substance.

C. A transverse section through the fetal head shows the lateral ventricles.

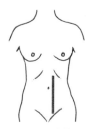

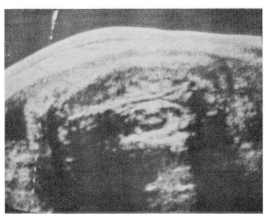

A

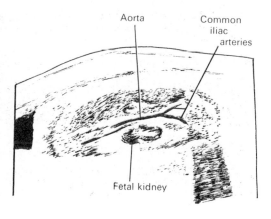

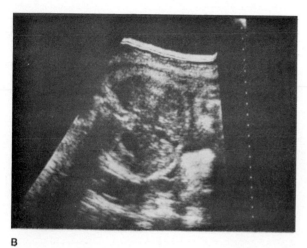

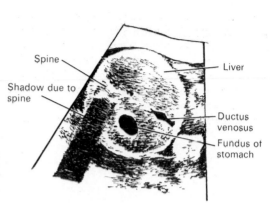

Spine

Liver

Shadow due to
spine

Ductus
venosus

Fundus of
stomach

B

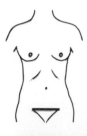

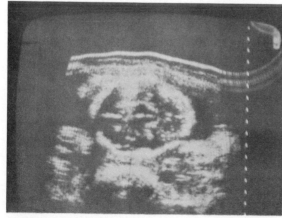

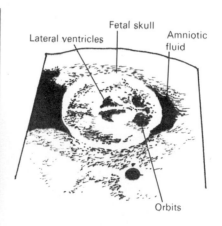

Lateral ventricles

Fetal skull

Amniotic
fluid

Orbits

C

10.16 The umbilical cord

The umbilical cord can be seen in most obstretic scans and appears as a tramline which is frequently in multiple loops. The upper figure shows a longitudinal ultrasonogram of a fetus in vertex presentation with an anterior placenta. The cord can be traced to its insertion into the placenta. The cord insertion has a significance while attempting an amniocentesis in pregnancies with totally anterior placentae. If the anterior wall of the uterus is totally covered with placenta, as seen in the transverse ultrasonogram (lower figure), it may be necessary to place the needle through the placenta to obtain a specimen of amniotic fluid. In this situation, it is important that the needle pierce the edge of the placenta rather than near the insertion of the cord, which has large vessels that might easily be injured.

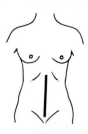

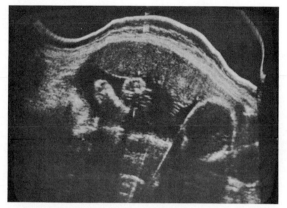

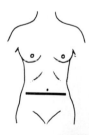

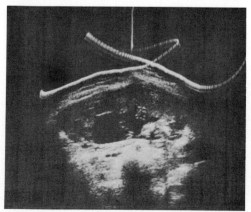

10.17 Twins

A. Longitudinal ultrasonogram of the gravid uterus 1 cm to the left of the midline (above) shows one fetus in vertex presentation. A further section 3 cm to the right of the midline reveals another fetus in breech presentation, with anterior and posterior placenta present. This is the most common arrangement for twins.

B. A longitudinal ultrasonogram through a gravid uterus reveals the fetal head of one twin separated by the amnion from the legs of the other twin, whose umbilical cord is seen.

C. Two fetal heads are seen, both in vertex presentation.

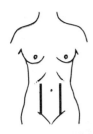

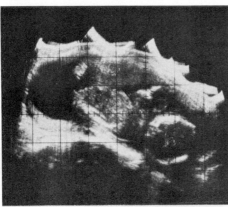

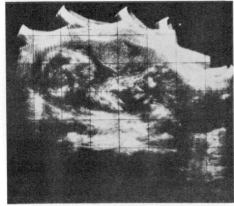

A

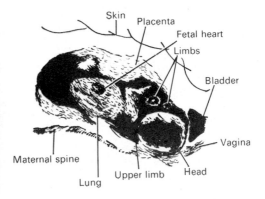

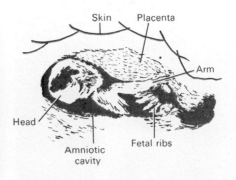

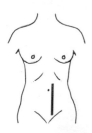

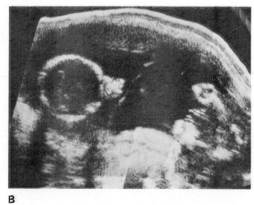

B

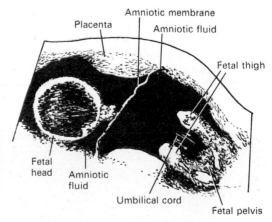

Placenta

Amniotic membrane

Amniotic fluid

Fetal thigh

Fetal
head

Amniotic
fluid

Umbilical cord

Fetal pelvis

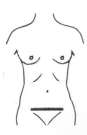

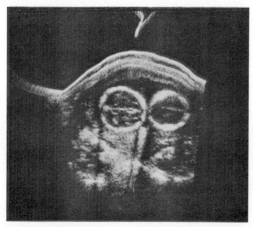

C

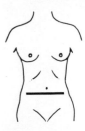

10.18 Twins with demise of one fetus

A. A transverse ultrasonogram through the gravid uterus shows two definite gestational sacs. The left sac shows definite fetal parts within it, while the right sac appears empty and suggests the possibility of fetal demise.

B. A repeat scan two weeks later shows marked diminution in the size of the empty sac, which is now undergoing resorption. These appearances are consistent with twins and demise of one fetus.

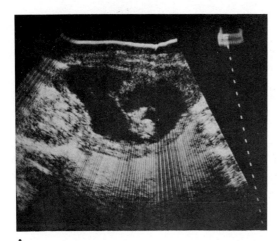

A

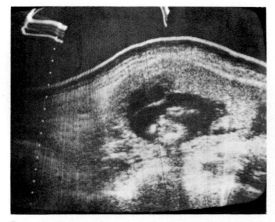

B

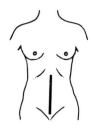

10.19 Migrating placenta

There is differential growth in the uterus during gestation with uptake of the cervix so that even if placentae appear to be previa in early pregnancy, there will be a relative migration of the placenta upwards. When the placenta covers the internal os, no significant change can occur; but extensive placentae are common which have one extremity approaching the internal os. A longitudinal scan of a gravid uterus at 19 weeks (upper figure) shows the placenta on the anterior uterine wall and a lower portion covering the internal os. However, the bulk of the placenta is clear of the os and such patients should be rescanned at 34 weeks to determine the definitive site of the placenta. The lower figure shows a longitudinal scan at 32 weeks' gestation in the same patient. The placenta is entirely anterior and there is no longer evidence for any degree of placenta previa.

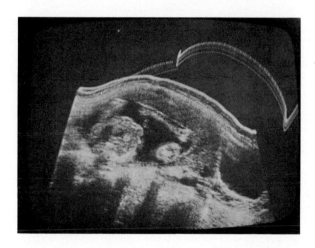

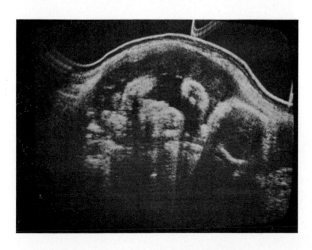

10.20 Placenta previa and placenta succenturiata

A. A midline section through the gravid uterus reveals the bulk of the placenta overlying the internal os, thereby producing a major degree of placenta previa which will not be substantially improved by any subsequent migration of the placenta. Frequently the fetus is found in the transverse or oblique lie.

B. *Placenta succenturiata.* One cotyledon of the placenta may be anatomically separated from the bulk of the placenta. Such appearances are seen in the longitudinal ultrasound scan, in which the separated cotyledon is seen in close relation to the internal os immediately posterior to the bladder.

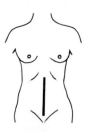

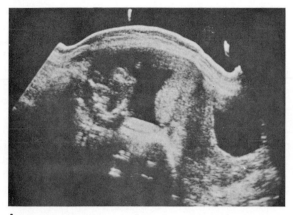

A

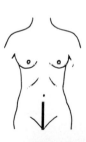

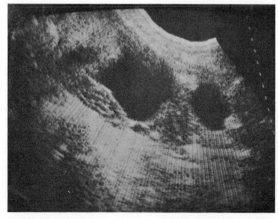

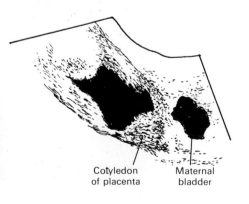

B

Cotyledon
of placenta

Maternal
bladder

10.21 Fetal position

The fetal position is very accurately and rapidly determined by an ultrasound examination. In early pregnancy rapid changes in fetal position occur which may cause the misdiagnosis of twins if the same fetus is seen in two different positions at different times during the examination. The availability of real time systems is particularly valuable to prevent this error. Vertex presentation is the most common fetal position.

A. A longitudinal ultrasonogram shows a singleton fetus in vertex presentation. The two chambers of the fetal heart can clearly be seen.

B. This is a transverse ultrasonogram showing the head and trunk in the transverse plane at the level of the umbilicus. The fetal lie is therefore transverse. The placenta is relatively poorly seen, owing to the shadowing of the fetal trunk. The head of the fetus is well flexed and both lateral ventricles are apparent. The lower limbs are seen in longitudinal section. In patients with persistent transverse lie, careful examination of the lower segment of the uterus must be carried out to exclude space-occupying masses which prevent version of the fetus. Such masses might include placenta previa, fibroid, second fetus or fetal malformation.

C. A longitudinal ultrasonogram with a single fetus shown in breech presentation. The fetal orbits, nasal skeleton and tooth buds can be discerned. Again, in persistent breech presentation, a careful search must be made of the lower segment of the uterus for any space occupying masses preventing version of the fetus. Alternatively, congenital malformations may predispose to breech presentation.

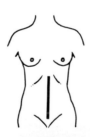

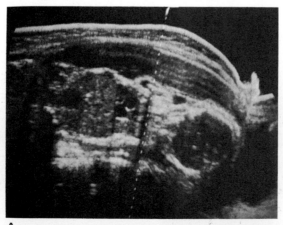

A

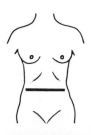

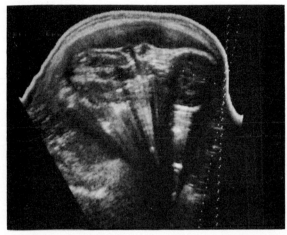

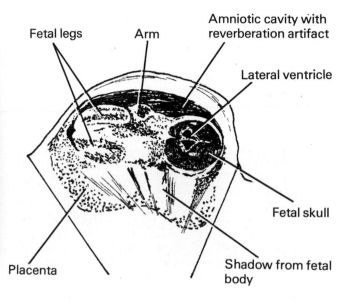

Fetal legs

Arm

Amniotic cavity with reverberation artifact

Lateral ventricle

Fetal skull

Placenta

Shadow from fetal body

B

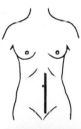

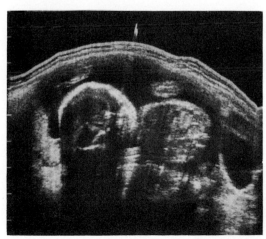

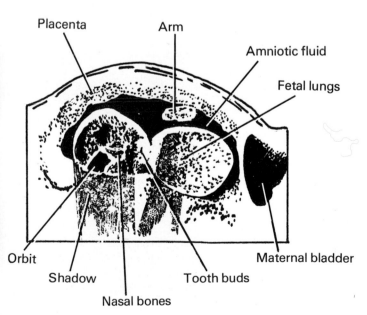

Placenta

Arm

Amniotic fluid

Fetal lungs

Maternal bladder

Orbit

Shadow

Nasal bones

Tooth buds

C

309

10.22 Fetal position—footling breech presentation

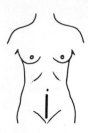

The longitudinal ultrasonogram shows the lower part of the fetal trunk and both lower limbs. One leg is clearly seen extended with the foot in close relation to the internal os. Such footling breech presentations are of particular danger in labor since the umbilical cord is frequently prolapsed, and this may result in fetal death. In this institution, footling breech presentation is an indication for immediate cesarean section.

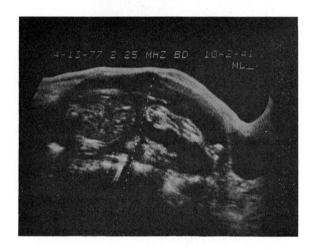

10.23 Missed abortion

Longitudinal (upper) and transverse (lower) ultrasonograms show the appearances of a missed abortion after 16 weeks of amenorrhea. There is no evidence of a normal developing fetus of 16 weeks' maturity and the gestational sac is in an advanced state of disintegration. Doppler examination reveals no evidence of the fetal heart which should be easily discernible at this time.

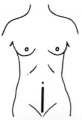

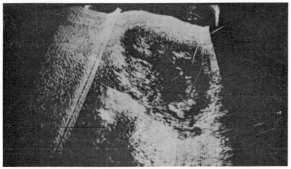

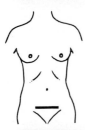

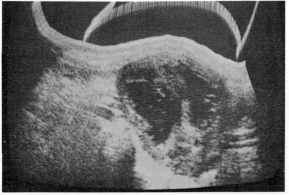

10.24 Hydatidiform mole

Hydatidiform mole presents characteristic ultrasound findings. These patients present with bleeding, suggesting a threatened abortion in early pregnancy, or with excessive enlargement of the uterus for the period of amenorrhea. The urinary chorionic gonadotrophin (UCG) is strongly positive. Ultrasound scanning shows the uterus to be filled with material with a consistency rather similar to a placenta. Definite irregular holes can be seen in the substance due to necrosis, forming cystic, grapelike structures characteristic of a hydatidiform mole. These appearances are well seen in the upper figure, a longitudinal midline ultrasound scan.

Hydatidiform mole with a normal fetus: Occasionally a hydatidiform mole may coexist as a twin with a normal gestational sac. This is shown in the lower figure. A normal gestational sac and a small embryo within it can be seen. Such pregnancies, of course, must be terminated, and the usual weekly follow-up on UCGs is carried out to detect the occasional malignant transformation.

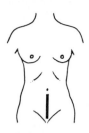

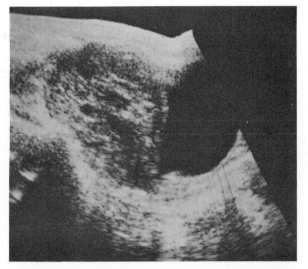

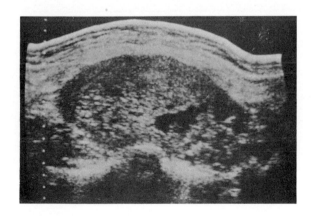

313

10.25 Polyhydramnios associated with multiple congenital abnormalities

This patient was referred for ultrasonic examination for a uterus that was larger than expected for her period of gestation. Transverse (upper figure) and longitudinal (lower figure) ultrasonograms reveal excessive amniotic fluid with marked fetal ascites, with which the fetal abdomen is grossly distended. Note that the placenta, which is seen anteriorly, does not have the thickened appearance of Rhesus isoimmunization. This fetus was found to have multiple congenital abnormalities, including gastroschism.

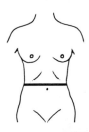

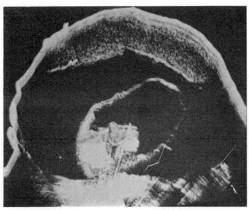

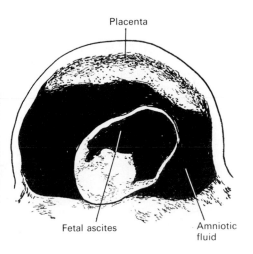

Placenta

Fetal ascites

Amniotic
fluid

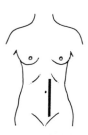

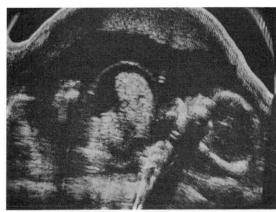

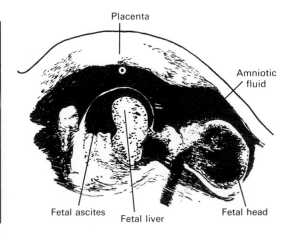

Placenta

Amniotic
fluid

Fetal ascites

Fetal liver

Fetal head

315

10.26 Rhesus isoimmunization

This gravida 5 was referred for ultrasound examination with a history of Rhesus isoimmunization of increasing severity, resulting in fetal hydrops in the previous three pregnancies. A longitudinal ultrasonogram (upper figure) shows a single fetus in vertex presentation and a posterior placenta. The placenta is very dense, thickened, and abnormally bulky. These placental changes are found in fetal hydrops due to Rhesus isoimmunization.

The transverse ultrasonogram (lower figure) shows a section through the fetal trunk; ascites are seen surrounding the liver and paravertebral structures. These changes indicate fetal hydrops.

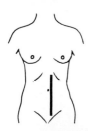

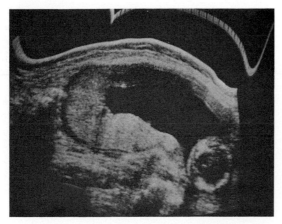

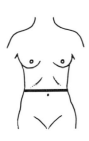

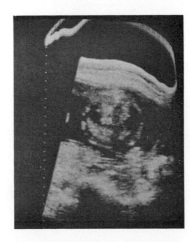

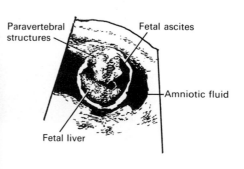

Paravertebral structures

Fetal ascites

Amniotic fluid

Fetal liver

10.27 Gross hydrocephaly

This 20-year-old woman was referred for ultrasonic estimation of fetal maturity at 20 weeks' amenorrhea. The longitudinal ultrasonogram (Figure A) shows a single fetus in vertex presentation. The fetal head is well visualized and the midline can be seen. On either side of the midline there is a cystic dilatation which represents grossly dilated lateral ventricles. Note that the uppermost ventricle has considerable artifacts due to reverberation partially obscuring the cystic contents. A transverse ultrasonogram (Figure B) shows the falx cerebri and the grossly dilated lateral ventricles. A thin rim of brain tissues is seen. A further longitudinal ultrasonogram through the fetal head (Figure C) again shows the dilated ventricles and the choroid plexus projecting into them. Between the head and the maternal sacrum, a portion of the placenta is seen. The size of the fetal trunk corresponded to maturity of 20 weeks, while the fetal head corresponded to 25 weeks. This pregnancy was terminated with prostaglandin, and a hydrocephalic fetus was delivered.

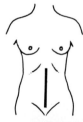

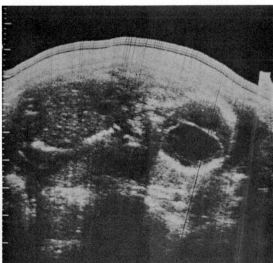

A

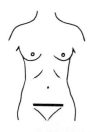

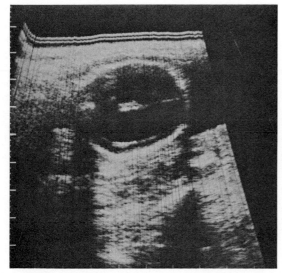

B

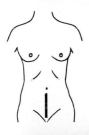

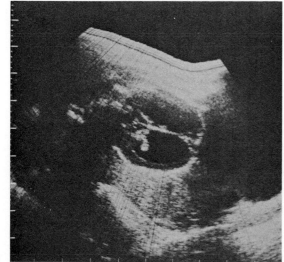

C

10.28 Anencephaly

A. A 36-year-old patient presented in her 35th week of pregnancy with polyhydramnios. A longitudinal ultrasonogram is shown, in which can be seen that there is a perverted development of the head which is consistent with anencephaly.

B. A patient was referred for ultrasound examination at 34 weeks' gestation to determine the cause of polyhydramnios. A paramedian section shows perverted development of the head, indicating anencephaly. This was confirmed radiologically and labor was induced. An anencephalic was delivered and died during birth. Anencephaly can easily be diagnosed by experienced workers using bistable machines, but this condition is simpler for the inexperienced to interpret using the gray scale technique.

C. This anencephalic fetus was diagnosed at 16 weeks and aborted. The superb detail of the fetal head permits a confident diagnosis to be made at this gestational age. (By kind permission of Dr. John Hobbins, Yale University Medical School.)

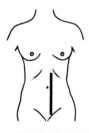

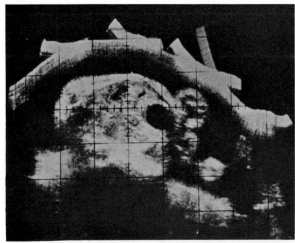

A

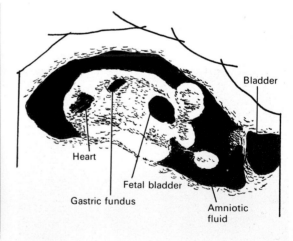

Heart

Gastric fundus

Fetal bladder

Bladder

Amniotic fluid

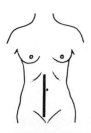

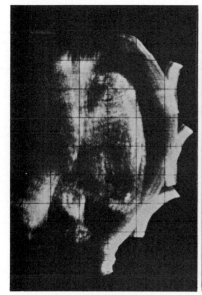

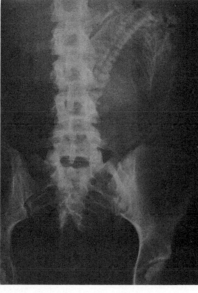

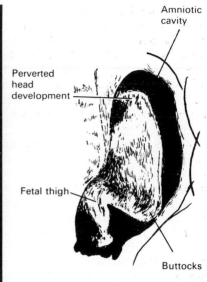

Amniotic
cavity

Perverted
head
development

Fetal thigh

Buttocks

B

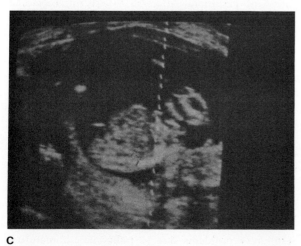

C

DETERMINATION OF BIPARIETAL DIAMETER

Rosie Silverman and K.J.W. Taylor

To determine the biparietal diameter, the gravid uterus is first surveyed to determine the lie of the fetus and the presentation. The plane of the scanning arm is varied until the scan is along the longitudinal axis of the fetal body and head. Next the plane of the skull and cervical spine is identified, since this compensates for any flexion or extension of the cervical spine. When scanning sagittally through the skull, a strong echo is seen which is part of the midline complex. The transducer is placed over this midline echo so that the ultrasound beam is perpendicular to it. The angle between the ultrasound beam and the perpendicular plane is the angle of asynclitism (Fig. 10.29A).

The scanning arm is then rotated through 90 degrees. In the most common vertex presentation, in which the initial scans are carried out in the longitudinal plane, the scanning arm will now be moved into the transverse plane at right angles to the lie of the fetus. The arm is then angled to the same extent as that determined by the angle of asynclitism. A transverse scan is carried out. The skull outline should be oval in shape. The scan is carried out so that the transducer is perpendicular to the long axis of the skull in this plane. The long axis of the skull is determined by compound scans of the skull. The position of the long axis of the skull is shown schematically in Figures 10.29 B and C for LOA and ROA vertex presentations, respectively. In scans in this plane, the anterior horns of both lateral ventricles are seen and the third ventricle is observed in the plane of the biparietal diameter (Fig. 10.29D). The midline echo, which is predominantly from the falx cerebri, should be in the middle of the skull, that is, equidistant from both skull tables (Fig. 10.29E).

If the midline echo is well marked but the third ventricle cannot be seen, the scanning plane is too high on the fetal head and the section is through the crown. If this measurement is taken, it will be smaller than the biparietal diameter.

If the midline echo is of very low amplitude, the lateral ventricles appear very small or are not seen, and a curved structure is seen on the posterior aspect of the skull, then the scanning plane is too low on the skull. A scan in this plane results in a section through the base of the skull and again is incorrect for the biparietal diameter determination.

If the shape of the skull is not oval (Fig. 10.29F) but appears round or foreshortened, the skull is being scanned obliquely. When such a round contour is seen, the scanning is not truly perpendicular to the longitudinal axis of the fetus. The correct lie of the fetus must be identified and the scanning arm again adjusted to be at right angles to that plane.

If the midline is identified but is not in the middle of the skull, that is, between the two skull tables, the angle of the scanning arm is incorrect. If it is closer to the inferior skull table (Fig. 10.29G), the angle of the scanning arm should be increased. If it is closer to the nearer skull table (Fig. 10.29H), the angle of the scanning arm should be decreased.

The various positions of the fetus are shown in Figures 10.29 J–M. They show the fetal head in those positions, and the correct biparietal diameter is shown on each projection. It should be noted that the biparietal diameter passes through the longitudinal axis of the head, which therefore should be oval. The correct biparietal diameter in the bistable mode is shown in Figure 10.29N. The nomogram for the biparietal diameter in use at Yale is given in Table 10.1. The nomogram was constructed from measurements of the biparietal diameter derived from the bistable oscilloscope screen. The bistable scan has some advantages in that the skull echoes appear thinnest and the measurement made is from the middle of each skull table or from the outer side of the skull table to the inner side of the opposite table. The thicker echoes appearing on the gray scale scan are not easily interpreted in terms of the bistable nomogram. Small differences in the nomograms constructed from different centers, notably those of Campbell in England, can be attributed to the small differences in the velocity of sound which are assumed by Campbell compared with that assumed in the construction of this nomogram. For the calibration of machines used in North America, the nomogram given here is appropriate.

It is technically easiest to estimate the biparietal diameter between 20 and 30 weeks of gestation since the head is easily identified and is relatively round at this period of gestation. After 30 weeks the biparietal eminences become more marked so that the precise biparietal diameter must be recognized; otherwise, there will be a marked inaccuracy in the maturity estimation. Furthermore, the rate at which the biparietal diameter changes after 34 weeks decreases to just over a millimeter per week so that small inaccuracies in the measuring process will lead to large discrepancies in the maturity estimation.

The biparietal diameter should be determined on every fetus before cesarean section to prevent the delivery of a premature infant. For this purpose, a biparietal diameter of 9 cm is considered adequate. Fetuses with a biparietal diameter of 9 cm seldom present problems with the respiratory distress syndrome, whereas those of lesser maturity may develop significant respiratory problems due to pulmonary immaturity.

Table 10.1 Nomogram for BPD using leading edge to leading edge (Yale) (*Courtesy of John C. Hobbins, M.D., Department of Obstetrics and Gynecology, Yale–New Haven Hospital.*)

cm	Weeks' gestation	cm	Weeks' gestation	cm	Weeks' gestation
		4.2	19.5	6.9	29.0
		4.3	20.0	7.0	29.5
		4.4	20.0	7.1	30.0
		4.5	20.5	7.3	30.5
		4.6	21.0	7.4	31.0
		4.7	21.0	7.5	31.5
1.9	12.0	4.8	21.5	7.6	32.0
2.0	12.0	4.9	22.0	7.7	32.5
2.1	12.5	5.0	22.0	7.8	33.0
2.2	13.0	5.1	22.5	7.9	33.5
2.3	13.0	5.2	23.0	8.0	34.0
2.4	13.5	5.3	23.0	8.2	34.5
2.5	14.0	5.4	23.5	8.3	35.0
2.6	14.0	5.5	24.0	8.4	35.5
2.7	14.5	5.6	24.0	8.5	36.0
					mature
2.8	15.0	5.7	24.5	8.6	36.5
2.9	15.0	5.8	25.0	8.8	37.0
3.0	15.5	5.9	25.0	8.9	37.5
3.1	16.0	6.0	25.5	9.0	38.0
3.2	16.0	6.1	26.0	9.1	38.5
3.3	16.5	6.2	26.0	9.2	39.0
3.4	17.0	6.3	26.5	9.3	39.5
3.5	17.0	6.4	27.0	9.4	40.0
3.6	17.5	6.5	27.0	9.6	40.5
3.7	18.0	6.6	27.5	9.7	41.0
3.8	18.5	6.7	28.0		
4.0	19.0	6.8	28.5		

10.29 Determination of biparietal diameter

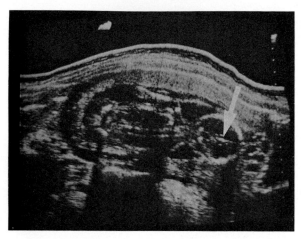

A. A longitudinal ultrasonogram of a single fetus in vertex presentation shows the position of the midline echo; an arrow represents the ultrasound beam perpendicular to it. The angle between the ultrasound beam and the peroendicular plane is the angle of asynclitism.

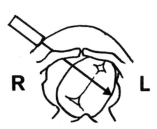

B. Schema of a fetus in LOA vertex presentation shows plane of scan to identify the longitudinal axis of the head and the position of the ultrasound beam through the biparietal diameter when this is perpendicular to the midline in the correct plane.

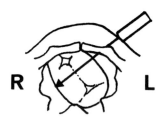

C. Schema of a fetus in ROA vertex presentation showing plane of scan to identify the longitudinal axis of the head and the position of the ultrasound beam through the biparietal diameter when this is perpendicular to the midline in the correct plane.

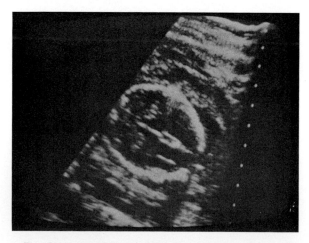

D. Cross section of fetal head in the biparietal diameter showing the anterior horns of both lateral ventricles and the third ventricle.

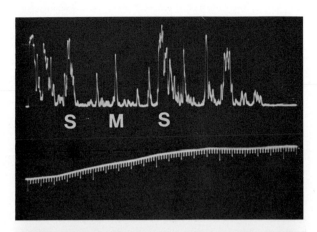

E. A-mode through biparietal diameter in the plane shown in Figure 10.29B showing the position of the midline (M), which is equidistant from the near and far walls of the skull (S).

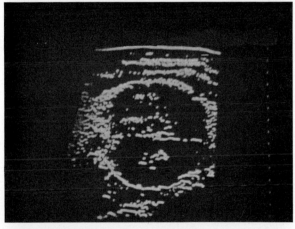

F. Cross section of fetal skull showing midline, but the scanning plane is not perpendicular to the longitudinal axis of the fetus. Note that this results in a rounded contour for the fetal head.

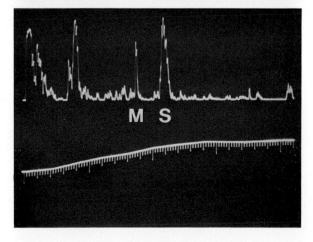

G. When the ultrasound beam is passed across the fetal head, the midline echo (M) is close to the inferior skull wall (S) and the angle of the scanning arm should be increased.

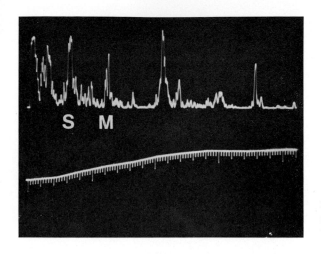

H. When the ultrasound beam is passed across the fetal head, the midline echo (M) is closer to the nearer skull table (S) and the angle of the scanning arm should be decreased.

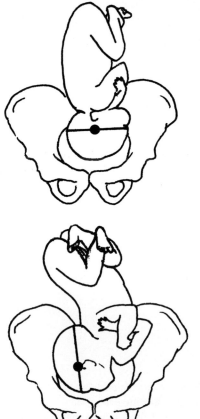

J. Vertex presentation with flexed head showing plane of biparietal diameter and position of transducer to obtain correct measurements.

K. Vertex presentation with fully extended head showing position of biparietal diameter plane and position of ultrasound beam for correct measurement.

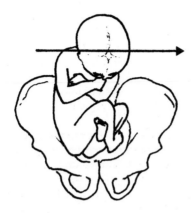

L. Breech presentation with flexed head showing position of ultrasound beam to obtain correct biparietal diameter.

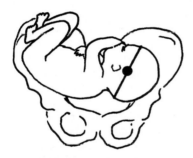

M. Transverse lie showing position of biparietal diameter and position of ultrasound beam to obtain correct measurement.

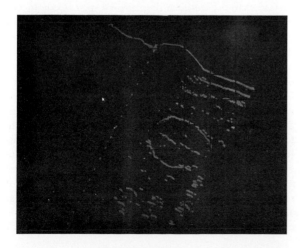

N. Transverse ultrasonogram of fetal head in bistable mode. Notice that the skull tables appear much thinner and it is easier to obtain an accurate measurement between the cranial walls.

11. Gynecology

GYNECOLOGICAL SCANNING

Ultrasonic examination of the female pelvis is largely complementary to the clinical examination or at times may have to replace or be supplementary to the clinical examination. The scan is carried out with the patient supine and with the urinary bladder physiologically distended to provide an acoustic window to the female pelvis. In the child or young adult in whom vaginal examination is difficult or impossible, the uterus and ovaries may be accurately localized by ultrasonic examination and congenital anomalies excluded. In particular, ovarian agenesis and bicornuate uterus or double uterus are apparent.

Ultrasound examination is also supplementary to, or may replace, clinical examination in the obese, in whom the presence of masses cannot be adequately excluded by clinical examination. In other patients with pelvic inflammatory disease, adequate pelvic examination may be prevented by discomfort to the patient so that again ultrasonic examination is required to supplement the clinical impression. In pelvic inflammatory disease (PID) the presence of partially cystic masses in the adnexal position is characteristic of bilateral tubo-ovarian abscess.

The differential diagnosis of palpable pelvic masses

Ultrasound has an important clinical application in the differential diagnosis of masses that are palpated on clinical examination. First, the size and shape of the uterus can be determined and one can accurately determine whether there is intrauterine pregnancy or not when there is a question of an ectopic gestation. The major contribution that ultrasound makes to a diagnosis of ectopic pregnancy is to visualize a nomotopic pregnancy. Although there is a very small chance of a twin which is ectopic, this is extremely unlikely. The characteristic appearances of an ectopic pregnancy are considered later.

Other causes of uterine enlargement may be diagnosed by ultrasound—most commonly, uterine enlargement due to fibroids. However, a word of caution is needed here, since fibroids usually appear as highly homogeneous tumors which return low-level echoes and frequently are irregular in outline and have irregular necrotic centers. These appearances in other anatomical sites usually constitute the characteristic appearances of malignancy and, indeed, it is impossible on purely ultrasonographic scans to differentiate between a fibroid, sarcomatous change in a fibroid, or even a carcinoma of the body of the uterus. These limitations should be recalled in any attempt to give a differential diagnosis of uterine enlargement.

Differential diagnosis of ovarian masses

The simple ovarian cyst can be easily recognized and accurately measured. Ultrasound examination allows documentation of the spontaneous regression of some of these simple ovarian cysts. Inspection of the walls allows one to assess the possibility of malignant change to form a cystadenocarcinoma. The solid teratoma of the ovary also presents characteristic, although not entirely specific, findings. In the diagnosis of a carcinoma of the ovary, again caution is necessary since a mass of fibroids extruded from the surface of the uterus, partially necrotic or irregular in contour, may simulate the appearances of bilateral ovarian carcinomas. Finally, ultrasound may be used to diagnose metastatic disease to the ovaries as well as metastatic disease from the ovaries to higher sites in the abdomen and the liver.

Endometriosis is a disease of modern times; it was not described in the literature until the twentieth century. It is characterized by extreme dysmenorrhea and by ectopic endometrial tissue which bleeds during the menstrual cycle and produces widespread blood collections both within the uterine tissue and on the serosal surface. More extensive depositions may occur in the gut, peritoneum, and even subcutaneous tissues. On ultrasonic examination, irregular blood lakes are found throughout the pelvic cavity, and this is characteristic of endometriosis.

Ultrasonic demonstration of fluid in the pouch of Douglas leads to an extensive differential diagnosis, and it is important that it is not immediately assumed that any fluid collection seen in the pouch of Douglas is due to an abscess. Most commonly, the fluid will be due to fluid in the gut; this must be differentiated by its characteristic contour or by repeat scanning after bowel motion. An ovarian cyst may, on some ultrasound sections, appear like free fluid in the pouch of Douglas, although more adequate scanning can prevent this confusion. Ascites may appear as fluid in the pouch of

Douglas, but this can be differentiated by finding ascites in other sites and also by moving the patient. In an ectopic pregnancy, finding a small amount of free fluid in the pouch of Douglas has an important implication—that there has been rupture of the ectopic gestation and that there is a hemoperitoneum. When fluid in the pouch of Douglas indicates a pelvic abscess, characteristically the abscess cavity is irregular in contour and often surrounded by high-level echoes from within the cavity indicating cellular interfaces in the contained pus; the fluid collection is constant and persistent in contour despite changes in the patient's position; and there is no change with time or bowel motion. Such appearances usually coincide with an appropriate clinical history and exquisite tenderness on attempted clinical examination. Thus ultrasound examination is the method of choice for diagnosing a pelvic abscess, although there are a number of alternative conditions which may simulate pelvic abscess and must be excluded by careful examination and observation.

11.1 Normal anatomy

The distended bladder, uterus, cervix, broad ligaments, and ovaries can be seen on ultrasound scanning. A longitudinal scan in the upper figure shows a physiologically distended bladder with the uterus lying posterior and inferior to it. The nongravid uterus is a pear-shaped organ, coning down into the cervix, which projects into the vault of the vagina. In the normal anteverted state of the uterus, there is approximately an angle of 90 degrees between the axis of the vagina and the long axis of the uterus. Transverse scanning of the uterus (lower figure) shows the body of the uterus; the broad ligaments and posterior wall of the bladder can be seen extending out from the lateral edges of the uterus. Almond-shaped swellings on the posterior aspect of this are the ovaries.

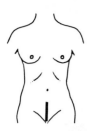

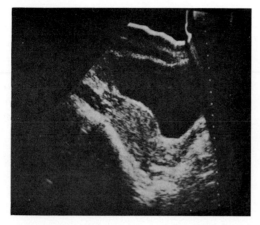

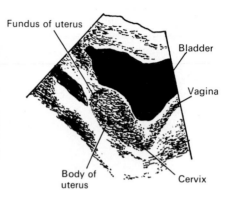

Fundus of uterus

Bladder

Vagina

Body of uterus

Cervix

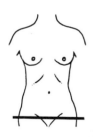

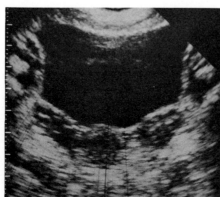

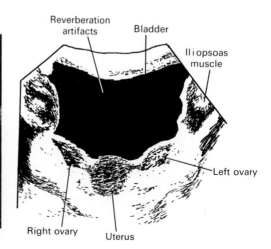

Reverberation artifacts

Bladder

Iliopsoas muscle

Left ovary

Right ovary

Uterus

11.2 Uterine and vaginal agenesis

A 15-year-old girl was referred for ultrasound examination to evaluate the contents of the pelvis. On general appearance, she had developed secondary sexual characteristics. Clinical examination revealed no evidence of a vagina, and rectal examination failed to reveal a uterus. The longitudinal examination (upper figure) reveals no evidence of a normal vagina and no evidence of a uterus. A transverse ultrasound through the pelvis (lower figure) shows a physiologically distended bladder with no definite evidence of a mature uterus posterior to the bladder. Careful transverse examination through the pelvis also failed to reveal any structures corresponding to ovaries.

This patient apparently has agenesis of the ovaries and structures derived from the Mullerian tubes. Genetically she was found to possess 46 chromosomes plus 2 X chromosomes, which is the normal complement for a female.

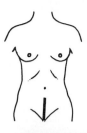

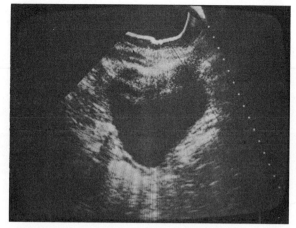

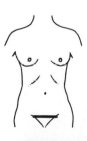

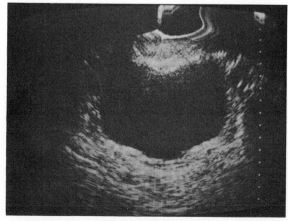

11.3 Double and bicornuate uterus

The female genital tract develops predominantly from the Mullerian duct system, and originally two separate ducts coexist which are destined to form the Fallopian tubes, uterus, cervix, and upper part of the vagina. Fusion commences at the caudal extremity—producing a single vagina, single cervix, and single uterus, but leaving separate Fallopian tubes. Various degrees of malfusion lead to a bicornuate uterus. Figure A is a longitudinal scan showing a cornual gestation in one cornu of a bicornuate uterus. The transverse scan (Figure B) shows the placenta in one cornu, while the other is empty. Major degrees of malfusion lead to a double uterus, as seen in Figure C. This patient also had a double cervix, but a single vagina. Complete degrees of malfusion lead to double uterus and double vagina.

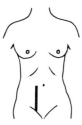

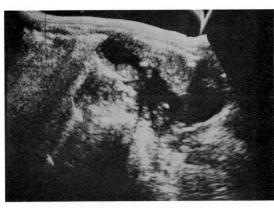

A

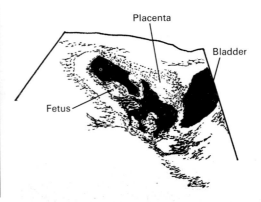

Placenta

Bladder

Fetus

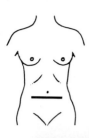

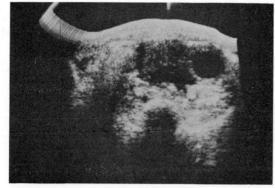

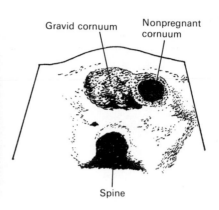

Gravid cornuum

Nonpregnant cornuum

Spine

B

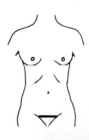

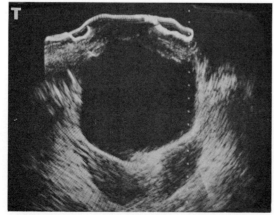

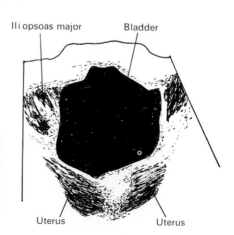

Ili opsoas major

Bladder

Uterus

Uterus

C

11.4 Intrauterine devices

A number of intrauterine devices can be recognized and localized by longitudinal ultrasound scans, including the Lippes Loop and the Copper 7. The Lippes Loop is shown in the upper figure, where the edges of the individual coils are seen. The straighter Copper 7 is shown in the lower figure.

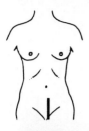

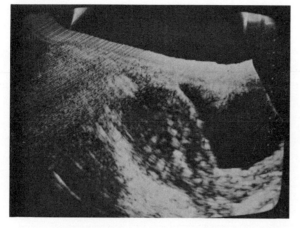

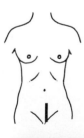

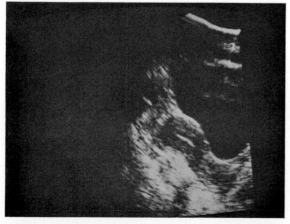

337

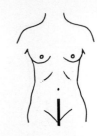

11.5 Pregnancy and IUD

This patient was fitted with an intrauterine device and presented six months later with a history of eight weeks' amenorrhea. Physical examination revealed an enlarged, apparently gravid uterus and she was referred for ultrasonic examination. A longitudinal ultrasonogram through the pelvis shows a gravid uterus lying posterior to a physiologically distended bladder. A small gestational sac is seen of eight weeks' duration.

A highly reflective linear echo is seen anteriorly, which is consistent with the presence of a Copper 7 IUD in addition to the gestational sac.

The coexistence of an IUD and a gestational sac is not unusual. Considerable difficulty may be found in locating the IUD in the increased volume of the uterine contents at a later stage of gestation.

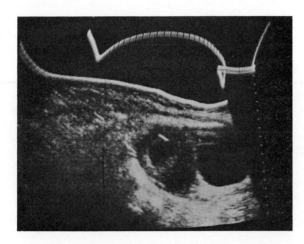
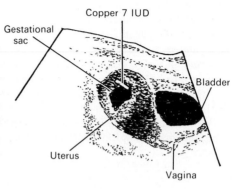

11.6 Tubo-ovarian abscesses

An 18-year-old black female presented with pelvic pain and persistent vaginal discharge for four weeks. The transverse ultrasonogram (Figure A) shows bilateral adnexal masses with the left larger than the right. The left mass is lobulated, has irregular contours, and is partially solid and partially cystic. The longitudinal ultrasonogram (Figure B) shows a section through the left mass which again clearly shows a central necrotic cavity. Such bilateral necrotic tumors could be neoplastic; but the clinical history of fever and purulent discharge, and the hemotological findings of leuko-cytosis, suggest an inflammatory condition. These appearances are consistent with bilateral tubo-ovarian abscesses.

A similar case is shown in Figure C, which is a transverse scan through the pelvis and shows a multi-loculated cystic mass in the left adnexal position in addition to a smaller fluid collection on the right. These appearances of tubo-ovarian abscesses must be differentiated from the simpler, but equally common, multi-loculated cystadenomas of the ovary.

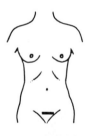

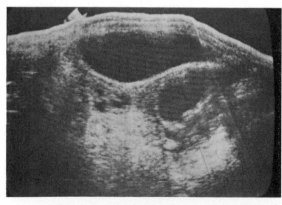

A

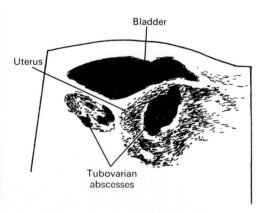

Bladder

Uterus

Tubovarian abscesses

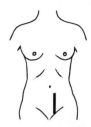

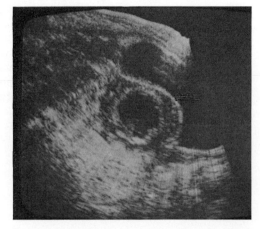

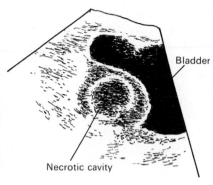

Bladder

Necrotic cavity

B

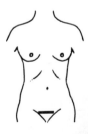

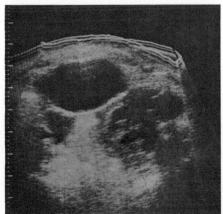

C

11.7 Uterine fibroid

This longitudinal scan (upper figure) shows a supra-cervical mass which is homogeneous in consistency, returning low echoes from the normal myometrium seen anterior and superior to it. The mass is seen on transverse scanning (lower figure) as a tumor continuous with the right side of the uterus. The mass is well encapsulated, and such appearances are consistent with a supracervical fibroid.

With current technology it appears impossible to differentiate between a fibroid and malignant transformation from the ultrasound appearances alone. Fibroids are frequently degenerating and appear partially necrotic so that malignancy is simulated. However, when these appearances are taken in conjunction with the clinical history, such as enlarging mass in a postmenopausal woman, it is possible to infer the probability of malignancy.

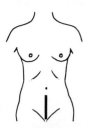

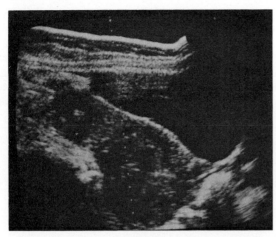

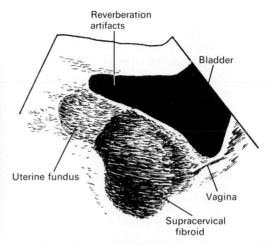

Reverberation
artifacts

Bladder

Uterine fundus

Vagina

Supracervical
fibroid

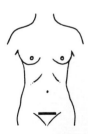

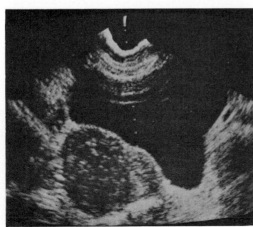

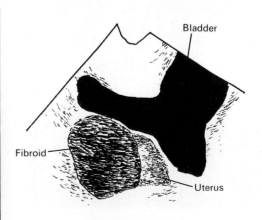

Bladder

Fibroid

Uterus

11.8 Uterine fibroid and early gestation

A. These transverse (upper) and longitudinal (lower) scans show a large anterior fibroid coinciding with a normal gestation. The gestational sac is seen posteriorly and is normal, whereas the fibroid appears as a homogeneous area arising from the anterior uterine wall with scattered internal echoes.

B. A transverse ultrasonogram through the fundus of the uterus shows a large fibroid mass with multiple fine high-level echoes, suggesting calcification. The right side of the uterine fundus shows a well-formed gestational sac containing fetal echoes.

Fibroids characteristically appear as more homogeneous areas than the normal myometrium. However, high level echoes are seen when there is calcification within the fibroid. Since fibroids frequently degenerate, irregular necrotic areas are often seen; these appearances may simulate malignant transformation.

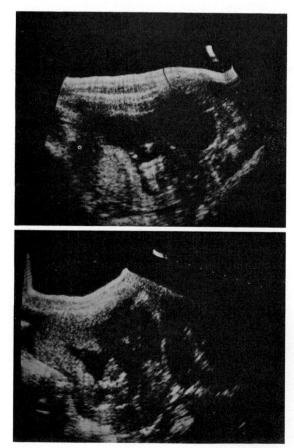

A

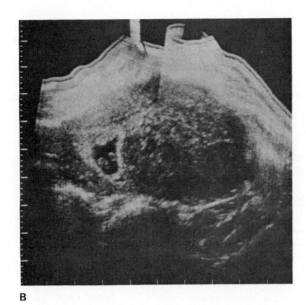

B

11.9 Ectopic gestation

A. This longitudinal ultrasonogram through the pelvis reveals an enlarged uterus, apparently due to a decidual reaction without definite evidence of a gestational sac. Posterior to the uterus in the pouch of Douglas is seen a cystic mass 3.5 cm in diameter.

B. and C. Transverse ultrasonograms through the pelvis 4 and 5 cm, respectively, above the symphysis pubis show a decidual reaction in the enlarged uterus but no evidence of a gestational sac. Again, a predominantly cystic mass is seen posterior to the uterus.

This patient presented with seven weeks' amenorrhea and investigations revealed a positive UCG. The major contribution that ultrasound makes to the diagnosis is the failure to demonstrate a normal intrauterine pregnancy, whereas a decidual reaction is observed. The cystic lesion could be a small lutein cyst, or it could be a hematoma surrounding the ectopic gestation.

Evidence for a small amount of free fluid in the pouch of Douglas is important, since the most probable cause is free blood in the peritoneum and this implies rupture of the ectopic gestation.

D. In another patient presenting with pelvic pain, this transverse ultrasonogram was obtained. A definite gestational sac containing fetal echoes is seen in the right adnexal position. M-mode examination showed fetal heart activity. These appearances are diagnostic of an ectopic gestation.

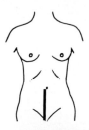

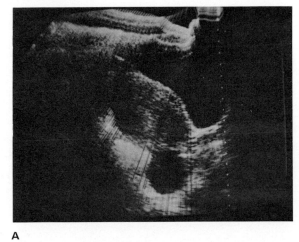

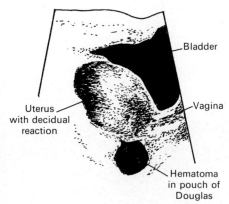

Bladder

Uterus
with decidual
reaction

Vagina

Hematoma
in pouch of
Douglas

A

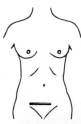

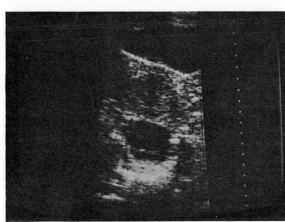

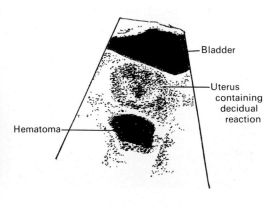

Bladder

Uterus
containing
decidual
reaction

Hematoma

B

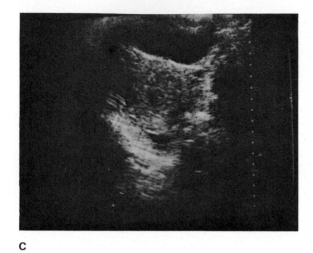

C

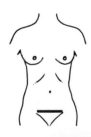

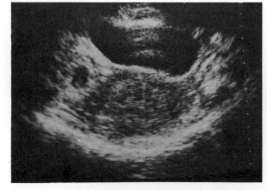

D

11.10 Ovarian cyst complicating early pregnancy

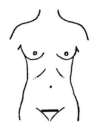

This 24-year-old patient was referred for exclusion of an ectopic gestation. She had a 12 week period of amenorrhea and a positive urinary pregnancy test. The transverse ultrasonogram reveals a gravid uterus displaced markedly to the left by a cystic mass arising from the right adnexal region. The pregnancy is definitely intrauterine. Although a twin ectopic gestation may coexist, this is highly improbable statistically, so that the finding of a normal intrauterine gestation is valuable evidence when an ectopic pregnancy is clinically considered.

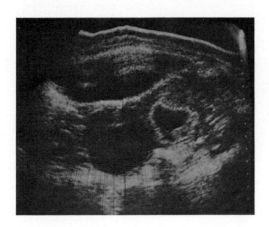

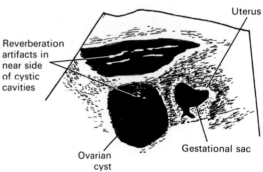

11.11 Resolution of ovarian cyst

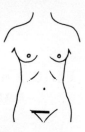

A 4 cm cystic lesion is seen in the left adnexal position on the transverse examination shown in the figure on the left dated August 3, 1976. Subsequent clinical examination failed to demonstrate this cystic area, and repeat examination, shown in the figure on the right dated August 30, 1976, indicates no evidence of this cyst.

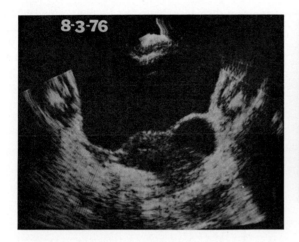
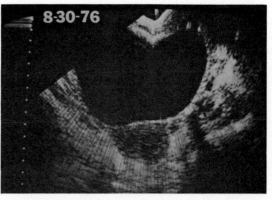

11.12 Ovarian cysts

A. Unilocular ovarian cysts

A transverse scan of the abdomen (left) and the longitudinal scan of the abdomen and pelvis (right) reveal a large single cystic cavity which fills the entire abdomen and pelvis and is consistent with a cyst-adenoma of the ovary. Note that there are small echoes within the anterior wall of the cyst; these are artifacts due to the sound beam "reverberating" in the anterior abdomen wall. Such anterior artifacts may be seen in the bladder, amniotic fluid, and gallbladder lumen.

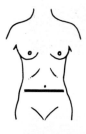

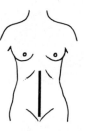

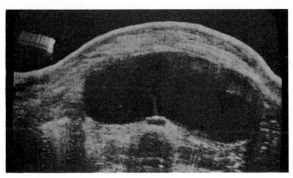

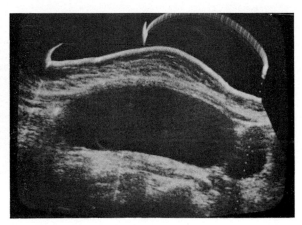

B. Multiloculated ovarian cyst

Transverse scans of the abdomen (left) and pelvis (right) show a multiloculated cystic mass. Note that a cyst fills the pouch of Douglas and displaces the uterus towards the left. The broad ligament and posterior wall of the bladder are seen between the cyst in the pouch and the lumen of the bladder. Ascites may produce similar appearances on a single scan, but differentiation can be made on further sections which reveal the cyst wall or septum. These appearances are consistent with a multiloculated cystadenoma of the ovary.

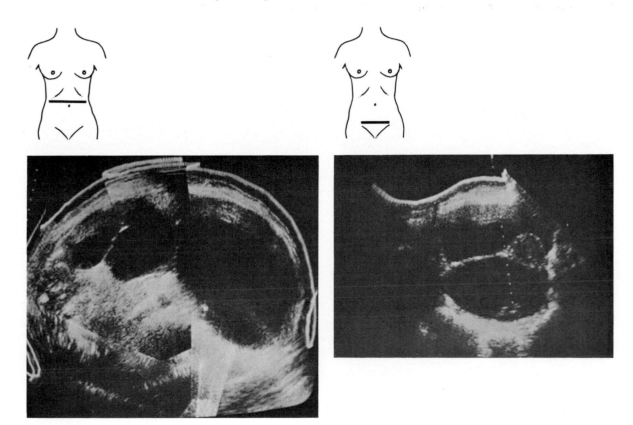

11.13 Cystadenocarcinoma of the ovary

This 57-year-old female presented with a large abdominopelvic mass and was referred for ultrasonic evaluation of the consistency. The scans show sections in the parasagittal plane through the right adnexal region. In the upper figure a predominantly cystic mass is seen with multiple septations and some evidence of low-level echoes within the cystic components. In the lower figure, there is much more evidence for a large solid component which is irregular in the level of echoes returned as well as in the contour of the edges. These appearances are most consistent with a cystadenocarcinoma of the ovary.

Laparotomy revealed a poorly differentiated adenocarcinoma arising from the right ovary.

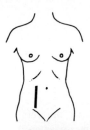

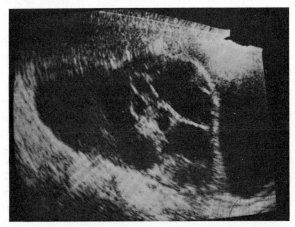

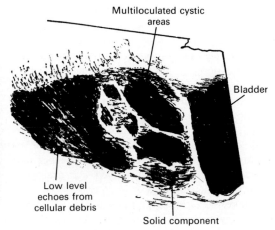

Multiloculated cystic areas

Bladder

Low level echoes from cellular debris

Solid component

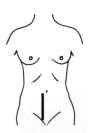

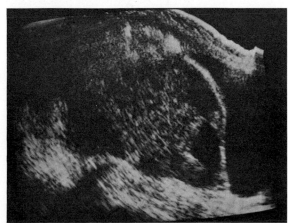

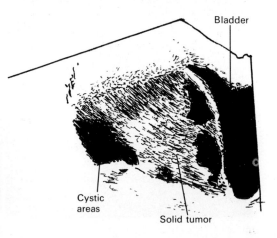

Bladder

Cystic areas

Solid tumor

11.14 Ovarian dermoid

A. A 30-year-old woman presented with a six month history of pelvic pain. On gynecological examination a cystic right adnexal mass was appreciated. The transverse ultrasonogram shows physiological dilatation of the urinary bladder. Posterior to the bladder the uterus is seen on transverse section. In the right adnexal position, a highly reflective and well-circumscribed mass is seen, which is 4 cm in diameter. The combination of a cystic mass on physical examination and a highly reflective mass on ultrasound section is virtually diagnostic of a dermoid cyst. These tumors tend to be highly reflective and highly attenuating to the extent that the deeper parts of the tumors may not be displayed. An example is shown in the following case.

B. Transverse ultrasonogram of a patient with an apparently cystic mass on examination. In the left adnexal position, a large, highly reflective mass is seen. This mass is 7 cm in diameter and displays such high attenuation that the deeper parts are inadequately displayed.

C. Paramedian ultrasonogram 2 cm to the left of the midline showing the highly reflective mass appreciated in Figure B. These appearances are virtually diagnostic of a dermoid cyst.

Dermoid cysts are interesting tumors in which all body tissues may be represented. Although commonly considered to contain bone and tooth elements, we seldom see any evidence of calcified elements in patients referred for ultrasonic diagnostic of dermoid cysts. Since they contain skin and sebaceous glands they contain fatty, sebaceous material, which is probably responsible for their scattering and attenuating properties. Of particular importance is differentiation of a dermoid from air in the colon. When a cystic mass is appreciated on physical examination but an anechoic cyst is not seen on ultrasound, the possibility of a dermoid cyst should be considered and reflected masses should not be dismissed as colonic contents. Repeat examination after bowel movement may be necessary.

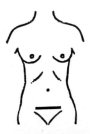

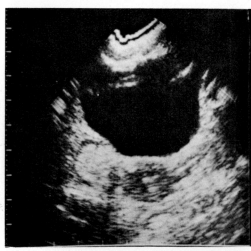

A

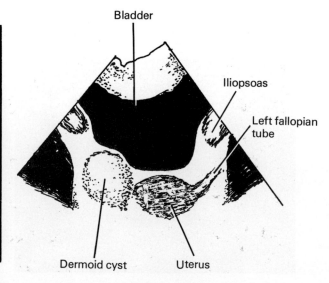

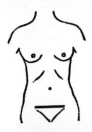

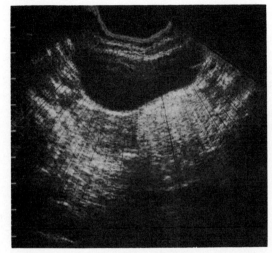

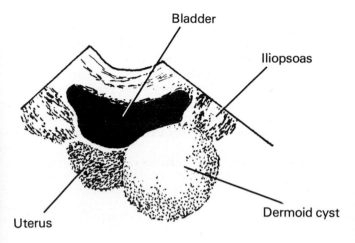

Bladder

Iliopsoas

Uterus

Dermoid cyst

B

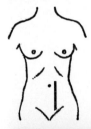

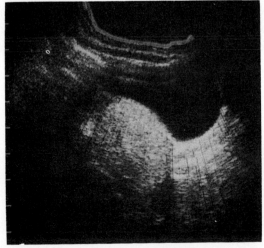

C

357

11.15 Malignant teratoma

A 14-year-old girl presented with a lower abdominal mass. Longitudinal ultrasound examination (upper figure) reveals a complex mass, partially solid and partially cystic, with free ascites in the pelvis. Transverse sections taken higher in the abdomen (lower figure) show solid tumor external to the primary mass. These appearances are consistent with an ovarian malignant tumor.

At surgery, a malignant teratoma was found with free ascites. Metastases were found in the omentum which histological examination revealed to be glial tissue.

Following surgery, this patient was treated with chemotherapy and the abdomen and pelvis scanned every month to search for possible recurrence. Four months after surgery a highly reflective mass was found above the liver, and this proved to be a peritoneal metastasis growing on the superior surface of the liver (see Fig. 4.40). Successful surgery was performed.

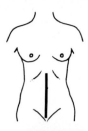

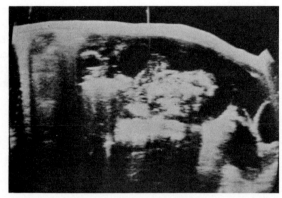

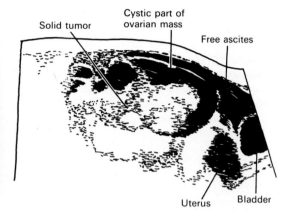

Solid tumor

Cystic part of
ovarian mass

Free ascites

Uterus

Bladder

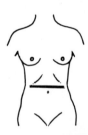

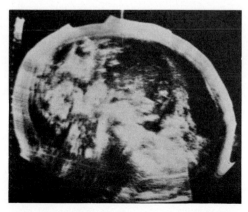

11.16 Malignant ovarian tumor

An 18-year-old girl had a malignant melanoma excised from her leg, but re-presented with evidence of widespread disease one year later. Chemotherapy was commenced, but she developed a neurogenic bladder and a Foley catheter was passed. On rectal examination, there was a suggestion of a palpable mass in the pelvis. Longitudinal ultrasound examination (upper figure) reveals an ill-defined mass lying posterior to the uterus while transverse examination (lower figure) shows a large solid tumor 6 cm in diameter, replacing the right ovary and causing the bladder to deviate to the left. This had the appearance of a metastatic tumor and accounted for her symptoms. She was treated with pelvic radiotherapy as a palliative treatment and there was marked improvement, with regain of bladder function.

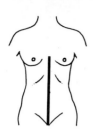

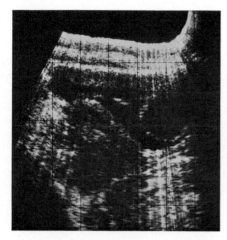

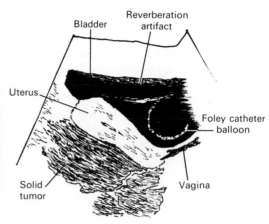

Bladder

Reverberation artifact

Uterus

Foley catheter balloon

Solid tumor

Vagina

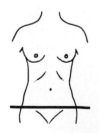

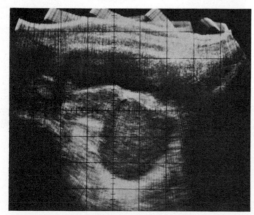

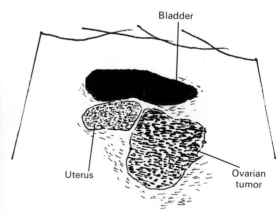

Bladder

Uterus

Ovarian tumor

11.17 Endometriosis

Endometriosis is a common disease of women in their third and fourth decades and is characterized by ectopic endometrial tissue which occurs throughout the uterine walls, on the peritoneum and ovaries or gut, on the rectouterine septum, and occasionally on more distant sites. Bleeding at these sites causes severe dysmenorrhea, tenderness, and dyspareunia. This may result in ovarian cysts which are due to resolution of the hematoma and are the so-called "chocolate" cysts or endometriomas. Such mature chocolate cysts are indistinguishable from other types of ovarian cysts if they occur, but are the manifestations of endometriosis. The transverse (A and B) and longitudinal (C) scans show cystic, irregular cavities throughout the uterine wall, and there are further cystic cavities on the peritoneal surface of the uterus extending out towards the ovaries. Widespread endometriosis was found on total hysterectomy.

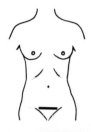

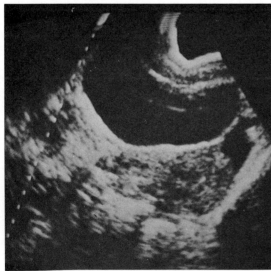

A

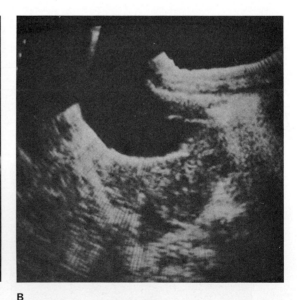

B

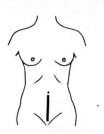

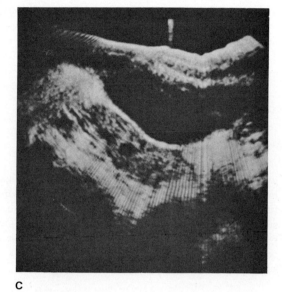

C

11.18 to 11.21 Fluid in the pouch of Douglas

Fluid collections are frequently seen in the pouch of Douglas and it is important to ascertain whether these are abscess collections, ovarian cysts, free fluid in the peritoneum such as ascites or blood, or contained fluid in the gut. These can usually be successfully differentiated by the appearances of the fluid collection and if necessary by reexamination on the succeeding day. These changes are exemplified in the following scans.

11.18 Pelvic abscess

A 22-year-old white female was seen in the emergency room with a history of increasing abdominal pain, nausea, and vomiting over a course of 5 days. On examination there was paralytic ileus, and a pelvic mass which was exquisitely tender. The differential diagnosis included a pelvic abscess due to a ruptured appendix, tubovarian abscess, torsion, and hemorrhage into an ovarian cyst. A transverse ultrasonogram (above) and longitudinal ultrasonogram (below) shows a highly homogeneous mass, indicating a fluid consistency which fills the pelvis. The contours are irregular and there are surrounding high-level echoes, suggesting the surrounding inflammatory reaction. These appearances are consistent with a sequestered purulent collection. At surgery a pelvic abscess was drained per rectum.

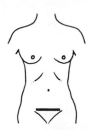

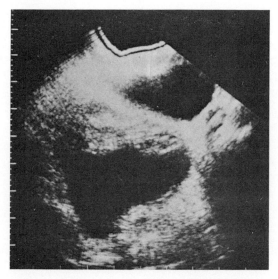

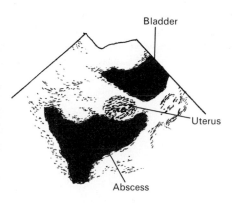

Bladder

Uterus

Abscess

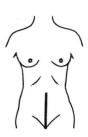

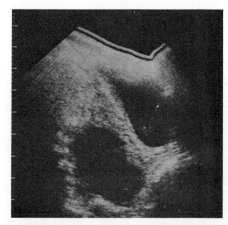

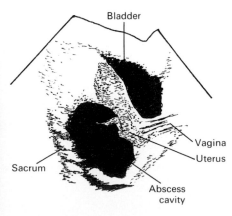

Bladder

Sacrum

Vagina

Uterus

Abscess
cavity

11.19 Ovarian cyst

An ovarian cyst may fill a pouch of Douglas and present as fluid in the pouch of Douglas, but this is well encapsulated and shows relatively thin walls. In many patients in whom fluid in the pouch of Douglas is due to an ovarian cyst, the transverse ultrasonograms will clarify the adnexal position of the mass. A longitudinal ultrasonogram (above) and a transverse ultrasonogram (below) demonstrate loculated fluid apparently in the pouch of Douglas on the longitudinal scan, whereas the transverse scan reveals that this is in the left adnexal position with the appearances those of a left ovarian cyst.

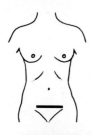

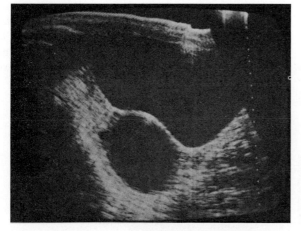

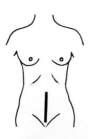

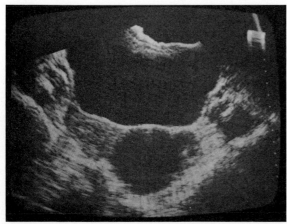

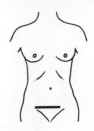

11.20 Fluid in gut

This transverse ultrasonogram through the pelvis shows fluid posterior to the uterus in the pouch of Douglas, but this is in fact contained in the small gut. On direct questioning, the patient will normally give a history of recent diarrhea, and the scan also demonstrates that the fluid is contained apparently in a lobulated tube. These appearances are highly suggestive of fluid contained within the small bowel. In contrast, free fluid in the peritoneum shows more rounded contour. The appearances of fluid in the gut can be confirmed by repeated examination of the patient on the succeeding day, when the fluid either will no longer be seen or will have changed in external contours.

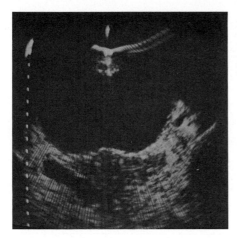

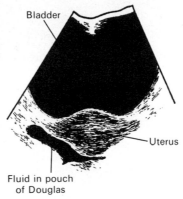

Bladder

Uterus

Fluid in pouch
of Douglas

11.21 Ascites

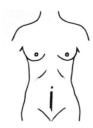

The appearances of free fluid in the peritoneal cavity as seen in ascites are shown in the longitudinal ultrasonogram (upper figure). The uterus is outlined by free fluid, and this fluid delineates the peritoneal reflections around the uterus. A change in the patient's posture allows this free ascites to move with gravity, but the characteristic distribution of the fluid collection allows the nature of this fluid to be easily recognized.

Smaller collections of free ascites as seen in this longitudinal ultrasonogram (lower figure) are more difficult to differentiate from other fluid collections in the pouch of Douglas, particularly those in the gut. However, a change in the patient's position, or repeat examination on the succeeding day, will aid in this differentiation.

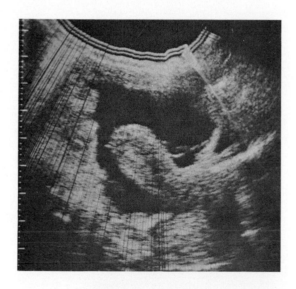

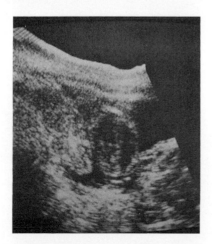

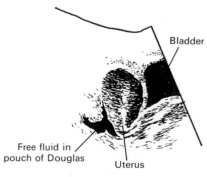

Bladder

Free fluid in pouch of Douglas

Uterus

12. The abdomen

12.1 Artifacts due to barium

Barium causes marked interference with ultrasound transmission and may produce confusing artifacts. This paramedian scan of the liver shows a dilated gallbladder with a highly reflective mass on its deep wall (upper figure). This mass appears to be partially within the lumen of the gallbladder. Note a definite acoustic shadow posterior to the reflective mass indicating high attenuation within the mass. These appearances may be confused with gallstones but, in fact, are due to barium in the gut. The presence of highly reflective masses outside the gallbladder permits correct interpretation. Note that in the lower figure there are multiple reverberations at the barium interface, suggesting a large discontinuity of acoustic impedance. Ultrasound examination should be carried out before barium studies or purgation should be undertaken after barium examinations.

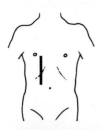

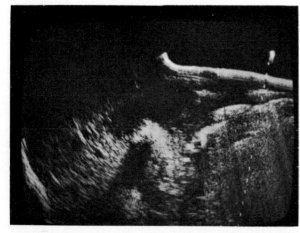

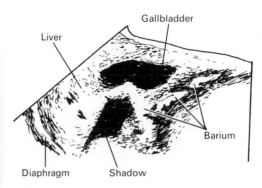

Liver

Gallbladder

Diaphragm

Shadow

Barium

upper

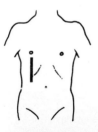

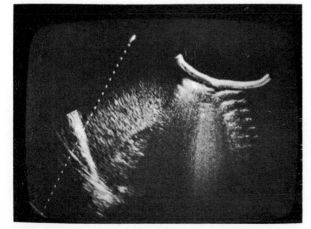

lower

12.2 Para-aortic lymphadenopathy

This 60-year-old female was known to suffer with chronic lymphatic leukemia for four years, for which she had received extensive chemotherapy. She was referred for ultrasonic evaluation of the upper abdomen.

A transverse scan immediately below the xiphisternum (Figure A) shows the prevertebral vessels, including a large splenic vein joining the superior mesenteric vein to form the portal vein, the superior mesenteric artery, left renal vein, and aorta. Anterior to these vessels, lobulated homogeneous masses are seen.

A hemisection through the right side of the abdomen at this level (Figure B) shows the right kidney again with a large lobulated mass anterior to it, consistent with para-aortic lymphadenopathy. These appearances are confirmed on the longitudinal scan 2 cm to the left of the midline (Figure C), which shows lobulated masses anterior to the superior mesenteric vessels.

Note that these masses are close to the pancreas and must be differentiated from a mass of pancreatic origin. These lymphoid masses are too well defined to be a carcinoma of the pancreas, which usually has highly irregular contours and shows evidence of local invasion. Chronic pancreatitis has not been observed to present this lobulated contour, nor generally to be of these dimensions. Para-aortic nodes may frequently be found to be posterior to the superior mesenteric vessels, which permits their differentiation from the body of the pancreas. In this case a more anterior group of para-aortic nodes are affected.

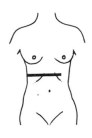

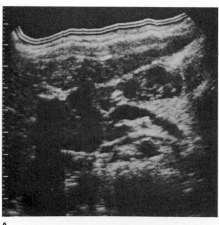

A

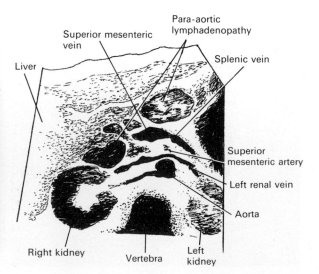

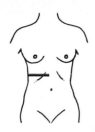

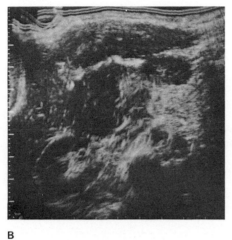

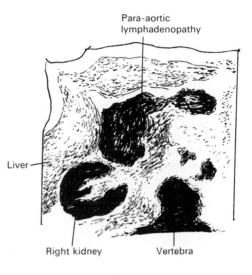

Para-aortic
lymphadenopathy

Liver

Right kidney   Vertebra

B

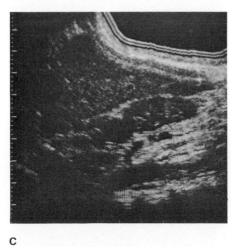

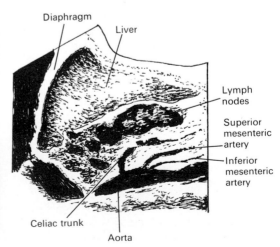

Diaphragm   Liver

Lymph
nodes

Superior
mesenteric
artery

Inferior
mesenteric
artery

Celiac trunk

Aorta

C

373

12.3 Para-aortic lymphadenopathy

A 24-year-old white male presented with abdominal pain and a mass in the midabdomen. Because of his alcoholic history, he was thought to have a large pancreatic pseudocyst. Upper GI series showed marked displacement of the central loops of small bowel with elevation of the antrum of the stomach. However, a transverse ultrasonogram (upper figure) shows a large, homogeneous mass surrounding the aorta. The longitudinal ultrasonogram (lower figure) taken 2 cm to the left of the midline shows, again, a lobulated homogeneous mass intervening between the superior mesenteric artery (arrowed) and the aorta. Such enlargements are almost invariably due to para-aortic lymphadenopathy. The uncinate process of the pancreas is also in this vascular space but most pancreatic neoplasms are seen anterior to the superior mesenteric vessels.

In this patient, clinical reexamination revealed a small tumor in the testicle and, at laparotomy, metastatic seminoma was confirmed in the periaortic nodes. (By kind permission of Dr. Bruce Simonds.)

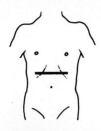

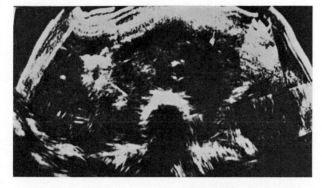

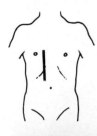

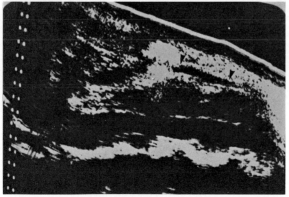

12.4 Retroperitoneal lymphosarcoma

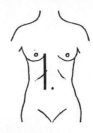

This 55-year-old female presented with a palpable epigastric mass which was first scanned by ultrasound at another hospital and was reported to be mainly cystic, suggesting that this was a pseudocyst of the pancreas. Repeat examination on admission to the Yale–New Haven Hospital showed a highly homogeneous tumor lying anterior to the inferior vena cava on the longitudinal section shown in the figure. Very low-level echoes are apparent, suggesting a highly homogeneous tumor such as a lymphoma or sarcoma. Careful examination of the interface between the liver and the tumor shows marked irregularity, suggesting active invasion of the liver and supporting the concept that this mass was malignant. Although percutaneous biopsy could easily have been performed, an open laparotomy was carried out which showed a malignant tumor of the retroperitoneum which was invading the liver. Histology revealed a lymphosarcoma. This case demonstrates how a highly homogeneous tumor, such as a lymphoma or sarcoma, may be mistaken for a cystic mass by inexperienced ultrasonographers. Although this tumor arose in the vicinity of the pancreas, carcinomas of the pancreas of this size are seldom seen and common bile duct obstruction would be expected. The marked homogeneity of these ultrasonic appearances correctly predicted the tumor type.

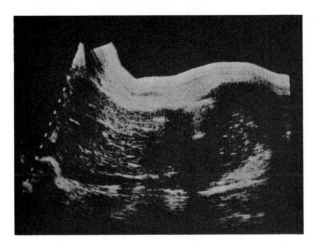

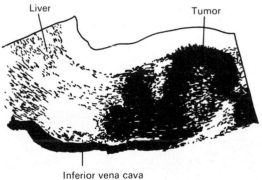

Liver

Tumor

Inferior vena cava

12.5 Retroperitoneal plasmacytoma

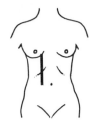

This 48-year-old female presented with a palpable mass in the right hypochondrium. A longitudinal ultrasonogram reveals a reniform, homogeneous mass lying below the liver and simulating a right renal tumor. An intravenous pyelogram displayed a normal kidney inferiorly displaced by a soft tissue mass.

Surgery revealed a smooth mass displacing the kidney inferiorly, which histologically proved to be a plasmacytoma.

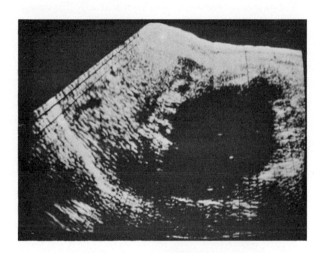

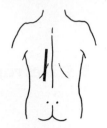

12.6 Left upper quadrant mass due to subphrenic abscess

A 20-year-old male presented with symptoms attributable to an islet-cell tumor of the pancreas. A 2 cm lesion was defined on pancreatic examination and excised at surgery. Two weeks after surgery, he developed fever, left pleural opacity, and leucocytosis, and was referred for ultrasonic investigation and localization of a possible abdominal abscess.

A paramedian ultrasonogram through the left upper quadrant from the posterior aspect (upper figure) shows the left kidney in longitudinal section and a triangular homogeneous mass between the anterior surface of the kidney and the diaphragm. The left hemidiaphragm appears abnormally flat, suggesting possible hemiparesis. These appearances were considered to be consistent with a left subphrenic abscess, and surgery was undertaken at which the abscess was drained.

Repeat examination three days after surgery shows the left kidney in longitudinal section with a small homogeneous mass near the lower pole (lower figure), which is the residual abscess cavity after drainage of the left subphrenic abscess.

Subphrenic abscesses are highly accurately diagnosed and localized on the right side and with an accuracy of approximately 90 % on the left side. Colonic content, fluid in the stomach, and air in the gut all make visualization of the left hemidiaphragm much more difficult than the right side, in which the liver provides a good acoustic window toward the right hemidiaphragm.

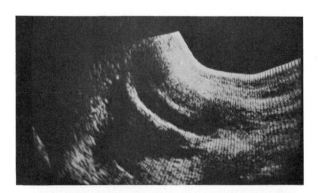

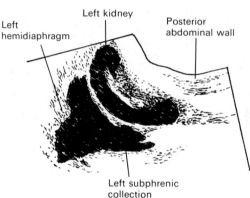

Left hemidiaphragm · Left kidney · Posterior abdominal wall · Left subphrenic collection

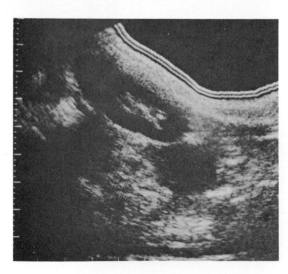

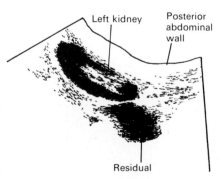

Left kidney · Posterior abdominal wall · Residual

12.7 Left upper quadrant mass due to stomach

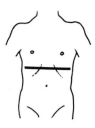

The upper figure shows a transverse scan through the epigastrium. There is a definite mass seen in the left upper quadrant which is continuous with the tail of the pancreas. This mass is predominantly fluid-filled and could be confused by inexperienced ultrasonographers with a pseudocyst of the tail of the pancreas. The possibility that this is fluid in the stomach should be investigated by altering the contents of the stomach. This can be achieved by aspirating the stomach if a patient has a nasogastric tube already inserted, or by giving the patient a drink of water.

The lower scan shows the mass immediately after drinking water; the whole of the cystic contents shows multiple gas bubbles, indicating that this is fluid in the stomach. Alternatively, a carbonated beverage may be given which is so gaseous that the stomach contents will be almost completely obscured.

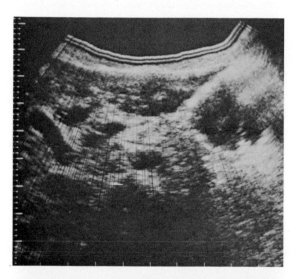

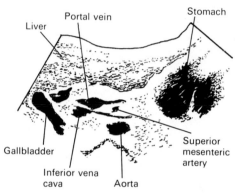

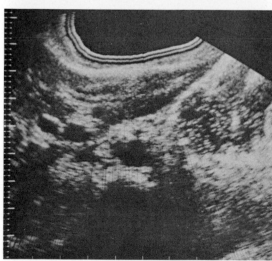

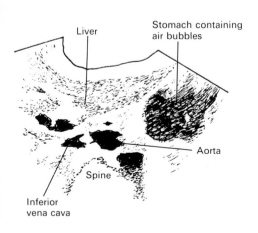

12.8 Left upper quadrant mass due to pseudocyst

This 46-year-old female was referred for a follow-up examination after a severe attack of alcohol-induced pancreatitis. No mass was appreciated on physical examination. An oblique ultrasonogram (upper figure) shows a large, cystic mass 6 cm in diameter in the left hypochondrium lying anterior to the left kidney and continuous with the tail of the pancreas. This is confirmed by a longitudinal ultrasonogram (lower figure). This shows the cystic mass anterior, but separate from, the upper half of the left kidney.

Occasionally such appearances are due to a distended stomach with gastric outlet obstruction. The patient can be given a drink of water or a carbonated beverage to see if bubbles appear in the cyst (Fig. 12.7), or a nasogastric tube can be passed and the stomach contents aspirated. The appearances here are consistent with a peusdocyst in the tail of the pancreas.

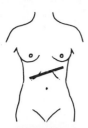

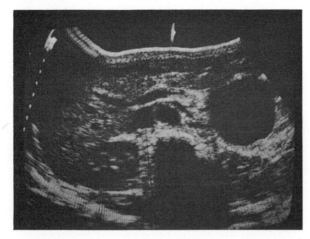

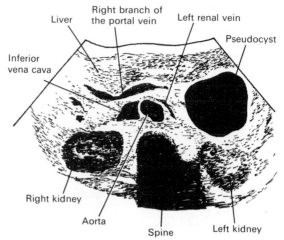

Liver

Right branch of
the portal vein

Left renal vein

Pseudocyst

Inferior
vena cava

Right kidney

Aorta

Spine

Left kidney

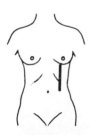

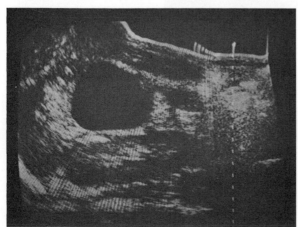

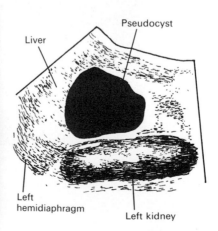

Liver

Pseudocyst

Left
hemidiaphragm

Left kidney

12.9 Left upper quadrant mass due to tumor

This 20-year-old female presented with a palpable left upper quadrant mass which had gradually increased in size over a period of two years.

A longitudinal ultrasonogram (Figure A) through the left upper quadrant reveals a large, well-encapsulated mass 16 cm in length by 12 cm in width. A transverse scan is shown in Figure B. The internal consistency shows irregular necrotic areas peripherally placed with high-level echoes more centrally located. The spleen was seen compressed posteriorly to the mass, and the left kidney was identified, displaced laterally. These appearances are consistent with a partially necrotic retroperitoneal mass such as a slowly growing sarcoma.

The high-level echoes from the center suggest a well-developed fibrous stroma.

Figure C shows the naked eye appearances of the cut surgical specimen which appeared most like a fibro- or liposarcoma. Electron microscopic examination indicated that this was a nonfunctioning islet-cell tumor.

The close resemblance between the ultrasonic sections and the cut surgical specimen shows the type of information given by ultrasound on any mass lesion. Although the final histology was unexpected, the differential diagnosis was similar for both the ultrasound and the gross pathological examinations.

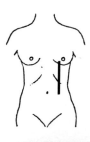

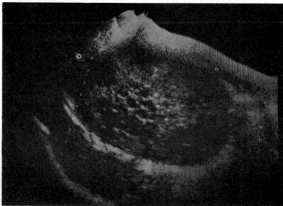

A

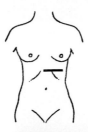

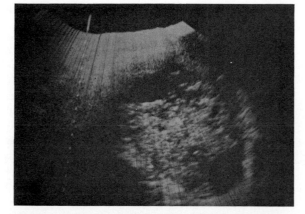

B

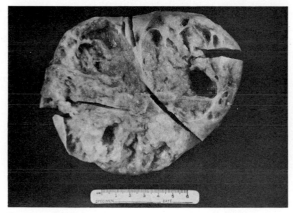

C

12.10 Right upper quadrant mass due to neurofibrosarcoma

This 11-year-old girl was known to suffer from neurofibromatosis. A palpable mass was noted in the right upper quadrant on physical examination and she was referred for ultrasound to differentiate the nature of this mass.

A longitudinal ultrasonogram through the right lobe of the liver and subcostal region (Figure A) shows a large irregular mass immediately below the liver. This mass is irregular in contour and echo amplitude and shows irregular cystic components characteristic of central necrosis. There is evidence of an irregular interface between the liver and the mass, suggesting local invasion of the liver substance. These appearances are characteristic of a malignant tumor in the subhepatic position.

The right kidney is displaced upwards by the mass and is immediately subdiaphragmatic in position. In this patient, who was known to have neurofibromatosis, the appearance of a malignant mass immediately below, and displacing the right kidney upwards, strongly suggested malignant transformation in a neurofibroma arising in the lumbar ganglia. At surgery, a neurofibrosarcoma was found. This tumor was only partially excised and

repeat ultrasound scans showed the residual tumor and were used for radiation therapy planning.

The response of the tumor to therapy was monitored by repeated ultrasound examinations. A sudden increase in the size of the mass necessitated a further examination. The transverse ultrasonogram (Figure B) shows a large cystic cavity within the tumor mass, and this was aspirated under ultrasonic visualization. Nine hundred cc of serosanguinous fluid were aspirated. A postaspiration repeat ultrasound examination (Figure C) reveals evidence for a highly reflective recurrent tumor mass in the liver substance, but little fluid remains. Repeated hemorrhage into the tumor area necessitated several aspiration procedures under ultrasound guidance.

The case history demonstrates the practical use of ultrasound in the initial diagnosis and clinical management of this young patient with a malignant tumor. Twelve examinations were carried out over a period of six months and the ultrasound scans record her clinical history. Especially in these pediatric patients, the use of a noninvasive and painless method of repeated examination is of particular value.

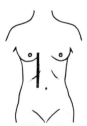

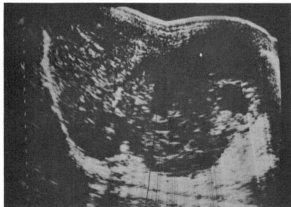

A

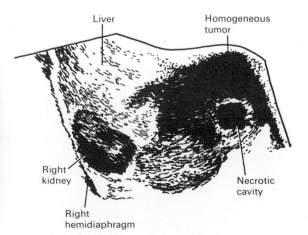

Liver

Homogeneous tumor

Right kidney

Necrotic cavity

Right hemidiaphragm

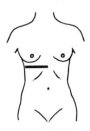

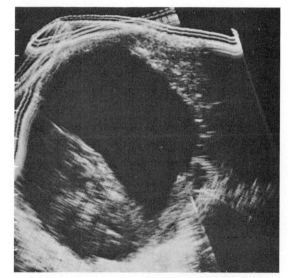

B

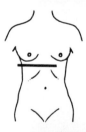

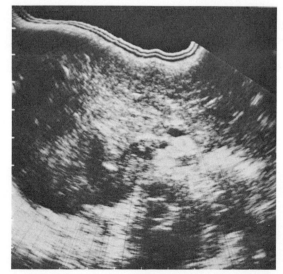

C

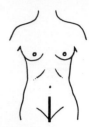

12.11 Normal rectum

The lower gut is not usually visualized due to its contained air, but this longitudinal scan of a normal female pelvis was carried out soon after an enema. The bladder is almost empty, but the normal uterus and vagina are seen. The rectum is seen lying within the concavity of the sacrum. The rectal walls are visible due to a small amount of fluid which is retained in the rectal lumen.

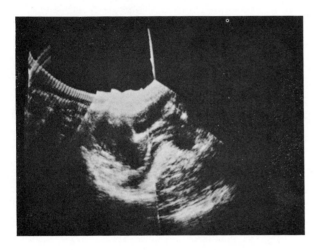

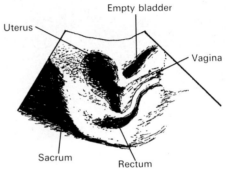

Uterus — Empty bladder — Vagina — Sacrum — Rectum

12.12 Carcinoma of the colon

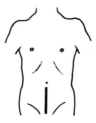

This 54-year-old male had a large palpable pelvic and abdominal mass which was known to be a carcinoma of the colon. He was referred for ultrasound examination to obtain a baseline for tumor size and to mark ports of entry for subsequent radiotherapy.

A midline section through the abdomen and pelvis reveals a large, solid tumor surrounded by free ascites. The solid mass contains many irregular, echo-free areas which are consistent with central necrosis. This evidence of irregularity in contour and level of echoes is strongly suggestive of malignancy.

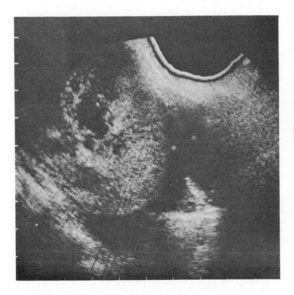

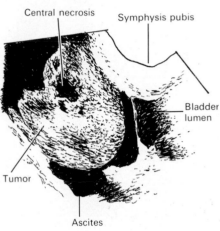

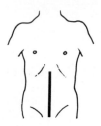

12.13 Tumor response to therapy

This 18-year-old male presented with a large abdominal and pelvic tumor which biopsy revealed to be a leimyoblastoma. On this longitudinal ultrasonogram, the tumor is seen filling the abdomen and the rectovesical pouch. A large cystic mass is seen superior to the bladder; this is a central necrotic cavity. Despite treatment, the overall size of tumor increased and solid tumor encroached on the cystic necrotic area when rescanned after one month.

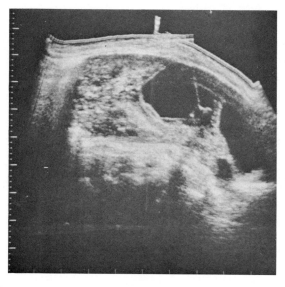

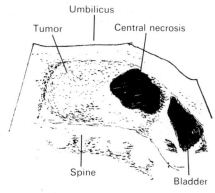

12.14 Histiocytoma arising from the urachus

This 13-year-old girl presented with a two-day history of fever and abdominal pain. On examination there appeared to be a midline lower abdominal mass just below the umbilicus. Intravenous pyelography and upper and lower GI series revealed no abnormality. A transverse ultrasonogram (A) and a midline longitudinal ultrasonic scan (B) show a highly homogeneous tumor returning low-level echoes but well encapsulated, situated immediately deep to the anterior abdominal wall. The appearances are those of a homogeneous mass, either an abscess or a tumor lying deep to the rectus abdominus muscle.

Exploratory laparotomy revealed a pseudoencapsulated urachal tumor locally adherent to the omentum. This tumor had cystic elements in it which were ruptured during removal. Histologically this proved to be a fibrous histiocytoma.

This patient was treated with radiotherapy and chemotherapy; ultrasonic examination six months later revealed a definite 2×5 cm mass in the right pelvis, although thorough examination by lymphangiography was normal. Two months later, the patient re-presented with fever and an obviously enlarging abdominal mass. Repeat ultrasound examination at this time shows that on both transverse and longitudinal scans (C and D), the entire pelvis is filled with irregular tumor material, with obvious areas of necrosis. At surgery this extensive tumor infiltration was confirmed and numerous peritoneal seedlings were noted.

This case illustrates the value of ultrasound not only as an initial diagnostic modality, but also for the follow-up of patients after primary treatment. Ultrasound demonstrated the primary tumor when all other investigations were negative. Of more importance, ultrasound also demonstrated recurrence of the tumor, but this finding was ignored in the presence of a normal lymphangiogram. A normal lymphangiogram may exclude disease in the lymph nodes, but extranodal tumor recurrence is best visualized by ultrasound or CT scanning. In this patient, in whom the maximum radiotherapy and chemotherapy had already been given, the delay in any further therapy resulting from the false security of a normal lymphangiogram was clinically unimportant.

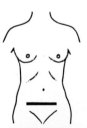

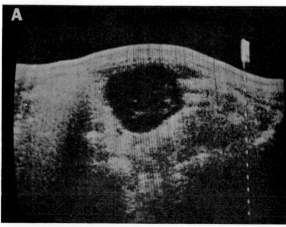

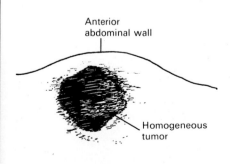

Anterior abdominal wall

Homogeneous tumor

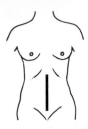

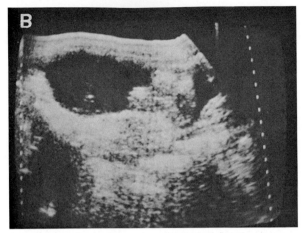

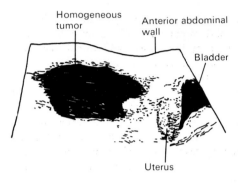

Homogeneous tumor   Anterior abdominal wall   Bladder   Uterus

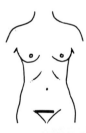

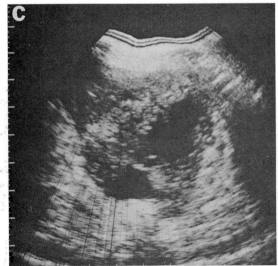

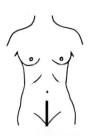

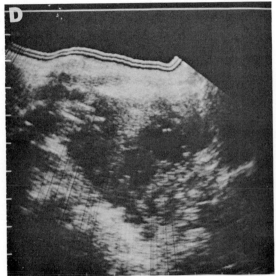

12.15 Abscess

This 18-year-old male was admitted with gunshot wounds to the abdomen involving the bowel and necessitating immediate repair. He subsequently developed fever and a palpable suprapubic mass. Ultrasound examination reveals a large cystic cavity on transverse scanning (upper figure) 4 cm below the umbilicus, while longitudinal scanning (lower figure) shows the same predominantly cystic cavity above the bladder. Posteriorly, debris is seen. Preoperatively, the differential diagnosis lay between a pseudocyst of the pancreas and an abdominal abscess. A sterile abscess was drained.

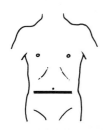

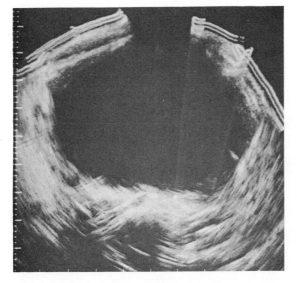

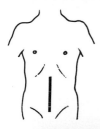

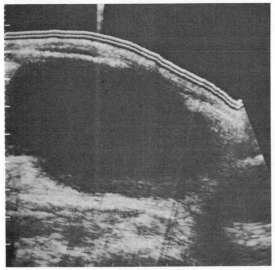

12.16 Retroperitoneal lymphangiomyomatosis

A 24-year-old female presented with abdominal swelling, and ascites was noted. A lymphangiogram at an outside hospital had demonstrated obstruction to the iliac para-aortic nodes with saccular lymphatic dilatation.

A longitudinal ultrasound section 2 cm to the right of the midline (upper figure) shows the liver lying anterior to the inferior vena cava. The prevertebral region shows multiple cystlike masses extending throughout the abdomen and pelvis. A pleural effusion is noted above the diaphragm.

A transverse ultrasonogram at the level of the umbilicus (lower figure) reveals similar cystic masses in the pre- and para-aortic position, consistent with retroperitoneal lymphangiomyomatosis.

At laparotomy, chylous peritoneal fluid was found with multiple diffuse saccular masses extending from the retroperitoneum to the right common iliac area. Biopsy of the sac wall and nodes at the root of the mesentery disclosed lymphangiomata. Treatment with medium chain triglycerides and low fat diet resulted in no recurrent ascites.

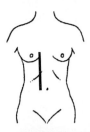

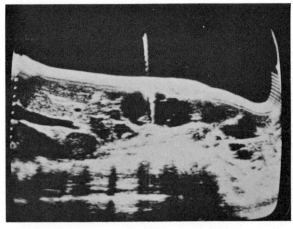

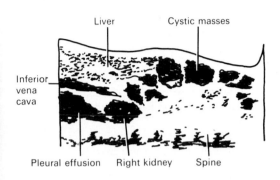

Liver   Cystic masses

Inferior vena cava

Pleural effusion   Right kidney   Spine

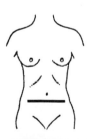

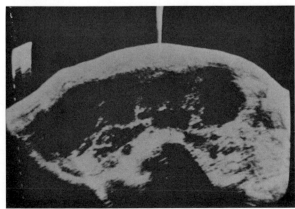

12.17 Ultrasonically guided liver biopsy

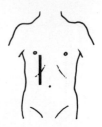

A 67-year-old male presented with a palpable mass in the right upper quadrant and ultrasonic examination revealed that this was a predominantly solid tumor continuous with the inferior margin of the right lobe of the liver and a central irregular necrotic cavity. An irregular border is seen between the liver and the tumor and the appearances are those of a malignant tumor invading the liver and displaying central necrosis. A simple cyst can be seen, in addition, on the lower pole of the right kidney.

A stereotyped liver biopsy procedure into the lateral aspect of the liver revealed normal histology. A repeat biopsy into the area indicated by the ultrasound beam (arrowed) revealed an adenocarcinoma.

Both ultrasound and CT scanning have been used to direct biopsy procedures of both the liver and pancreas. It seems most probable that the commercial availability of high resolution real-time scanners will greatly increase the number of such procedures performed. Using real-time machines, it should be possible to visualize the passage of the biopsy needle through tissue to the area of interest and to direct the anatomical site of the biopsy procedure.

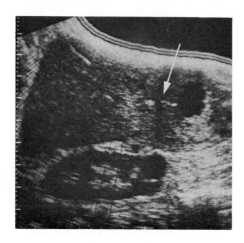

13. The thyroid

13.1 Thyroid scanning techniques

The anatomical position of the thyroid gland in such a superficial site produces both advantages and disadvantages for its ultrasonic examination. When the gland is examined by a contact scan, that is, with the transducer in contact with the skin, the initial transmit pulse produces a heavy echo which may obscure the superficial parts of the gland. Furthermore, the field intensity profile close to the transducer face is nonuniform and results in suboptimal resolution. On the other hand, the superficial site of the gland means that high frequencies of between 5 and 10 MHz can be used, although, since these transducers are generally driven by general purpose machines designed for abdominal studies, this effectively limits the frequency which may be used to 5 MHz. During the next 12 months, a dedicated "carotid scanner" developed at the Stanford Research Institute should be commercially available. Such a machine functioning in the 7-to-10 MHz range should be optimal for scanning the thyroid. Meanwhile, attempts to image the thyroid gland must be limited to the use of general purpose instruments; and in many community hospitals, this situation may persist for some time. Nevertheless, extremely useful information can be obtained, particularly to differentiate between cold areas seen on the nuclear scan due to cysts and those due to solid masses.

The thyroid gland can be scanned either by using a water bath or using a contact transducer. If a contact scan is carried out, most frequently a 5 MHz transducer is used with a 6 mm active face. This results in a collimated beam as shown schematically in Figure 1.5B.

In the more rounded female neck, such a transducer produces adequate scans and is also adequate for longitudinal scans in the neck. However, for the more angular male neck, technically adequate scans are extremely difficult to obtain and better results are obtained using a water bath.

Using the water bath technique, a plastic frame is made with a side limb which can rest against the bed on either side of the patient's neck. A simple frame connects these two side limbs, from which a polyethylene water bag is suspended (Fig. 13.1). This is filled with water and if left open to the air for 24 hours, the water soon becomes degassed. Patients do not appear to suffer discomfort from a depth of some 5 or 6 cm of water over the neck. The transducer is then moved in a simple transverse scan in the open water bath at a suitable distance from the skin to ensure that the thyroid gland lies in the focal plane of the transducer.

Technically adequate scans can be obtained by a 3.5 or 5 MHz transducer focusing in the range of 4 to 5 cm from the transducer face. This ensures that the target is outside the near field of the transducer and in the optimal focal plane.

One problem resulting from the use of a water bath is that there is low attenuation through the water bath so that the tissues are overcompensated for tissue attenuation. These appearances can be greatly improved by delaying the start of the TGC until the most proximal skin line, although a more elegant solution would be to trigger the TGC with the skin line echoes. The results of thyroid scanning are now considered.

13.2 Normal anatomy

This transverse ultrasonogram through the normal thyroid is a linear scan carried out through a water bag. The important feature of gray scale ultrasonography is that the glandular tissue of the thyroid is displayed, and the lateral lobes are well seen here lying on each side of the trachea. The trachea causes total attenuation of the ultrasound beam due to its contained air. Posterior to the lateral lobes of the thyroid the common carotid artery and internal jugular vein are seen lying within the carotid sheath. More posterior structures could be the vagus and sympathetic trunk. The strap muscles are seen anteriorly, while the sternomastoid is seen laterally.

The importance of displaying normal glandular structure is that carcinomas can be identified as areas which are abnormally homogeneous (blacker). In our experience to date, Hashimoto's thyroiditis may mimic a malignant process. Ultrasound examination displays the anatomy and pathology, while isotope examination indicates the functional aspects.

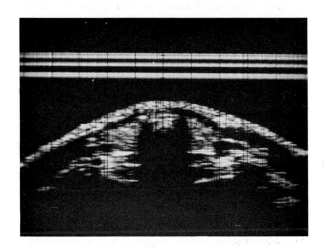

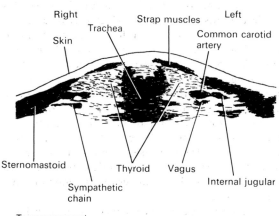

Transverse section of thyroid at level of C6-7

13.3 Cyst producing cold area on isotope scan

An 18-year-old male presented with a three month history of a painless mass in the right lobe of the thyroid gland. On examination, he was euthyroid and the mass felt firm. The isotope examination shows a relatively cold area (C). He was referred for ultrasound exam-ination to differentiate between solid and cystic con-sistencies.

A transverse ultrasonogram in the plane shown by the dotted line on the isotope scan reveals a completely echo-free area in the right lobe of the thyroid, and this is clearly a cystic swelling.

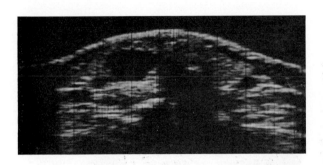

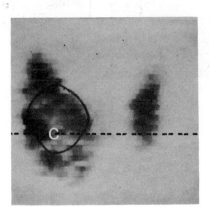

13.4 Adenoma

This 25-year-old patient was referred with a palpable mass in the right lobe of the thyroid which failed to take up radioactive iodine. The ultrasound was carried out through a water bath. A transverse section across the neck (Figure A) shows marked enlargement of the right lobe of the thyroid, but normal glandular tissue is seen throughout. The vascular bundle appears to be displayed laterally compared with the normal left side of the thyroid.

In a longitudinal section (Figure B) the solid mass is seen lying anterior to the common carotid artery, and again normal glandular tissue is seen throughout the gland. There is no evidence of any cystic component. The appearances are consistent with an adenoma of the thyroid gland.

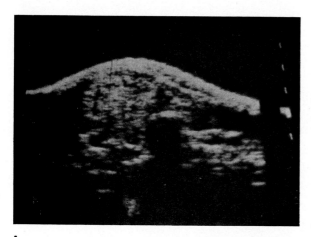

A

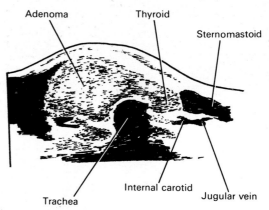

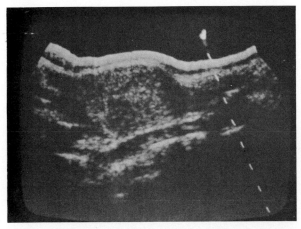

B

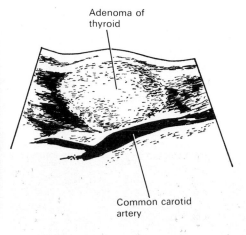

Adenoma of
thyroid

Common carotid
artery

13.5 Toxic goiter

A 28-year-old female presented with symptoms of thyrotoxicosis. The ^{131}I scan shows equal uptake in both lobes of the thyroid. A transverse ultrasonogram (upper figure) in the plane marked AA on the isotope scan shows both lobes of the thyroid gland, which are symmetrically enlarged and surround the trachea (T). The internal carotid artery and jugular vein are seen posterior to the lateral lobe of the thyroid. The skin and investing layer of the deep cervical fascia are separately differentiated. A further transverse ultrasonogram (lower figure) in the plane marked BB on the isotope scan shows a small cystic area (C) in the right lobe of the thyroid which, in retrospect, can be seen as an ill-defined cold area on the isotope scan.

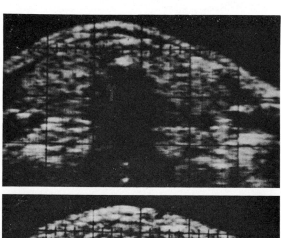

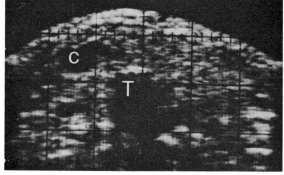

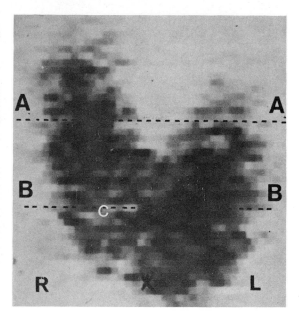

13.6 Lymphosarcoma

A 63-year-old male presented with a three-month history of an enlarging lump in the left side of the neck. An ^{131}Iodine scan shows that the mass fails to concentrate the isotope. The transverse ultrasonogram shows an abnormally homogeneous mass consistent with malignant replacement. This was confirmed at surgery and the histology proved to be lymphosarcoma.

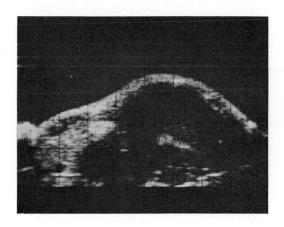

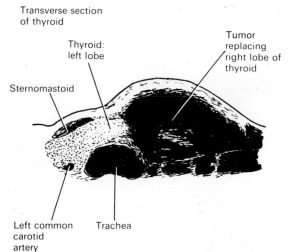

Transverse section of thyroid

Thyroid: left lobe

Tumor replacing right lobe of thyroid

Sternomastoid

Left common carotid artery

Trachea

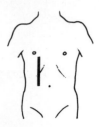

14. The thorax

14.1 Pleural effusion

The chest radiograph shows a patient with both consolidation and a pleural effusion at the right base. There is an opacity in the left upper lobe which was considered to be a bronchogenic carcinoma. Parasagittal ultrasonograms in expiration (upper figure) and inspiration (lower figure) show sections through normal liver, diaphragm, pleural effusion, and lung. The base of the lung must be consolidated, since aerated lung does not transmit ultrasound of this frequency. Comparison of the two scans shows that the diaphragm has descended and there has been widening of the costophrenic angle with inspiration. Thus the excursion of the diaphragm can be confirmed and measured. The normal appearance of the liver excludes a subphrenic collection and the absence of echoes from the pleural cavity confirms the presence of an effusion.

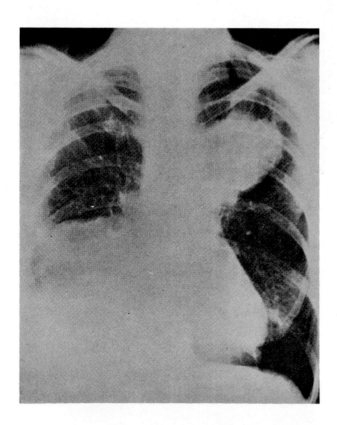

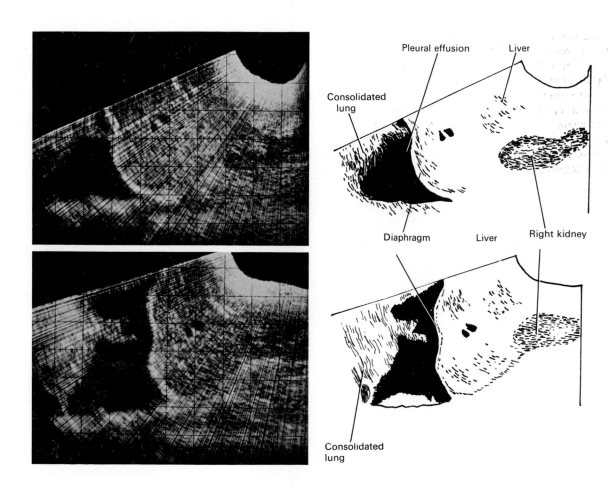

405

14.2 Pleural empyema

This 4-year-old girl had staphylococcal pneumonia which resulted in a persistent fever, leucocytosis to 23 000 mm^3, and persistent right lung field opacity. No fluid was apparent on decubitus films. She was referred to ultrasound to further investigate the cause of her pleural opacity and, in particular, to rule out an empyema. The child was very active during this procedure. A longitudinal scan (upper figure) through the liver reveals the right hemidiaphragm, which moved with respiration, and definite fluid in the costophrenic angle above the diaphragm below consolidated right lung. Further scanning on the anterior and posterior aspects of the thorax (lower figure) shows the right kidney with homogeneous material above the kidney in the right hemithorax, but definite echoes are seen in this fluid, indicating cellular debris. Such findings suggest an empyema. A needle was inserted into a pocket of fluid under ultrasound visualization and 1 pint of pus was aspirated.

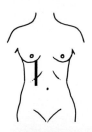

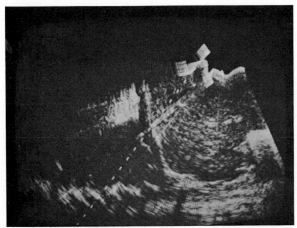

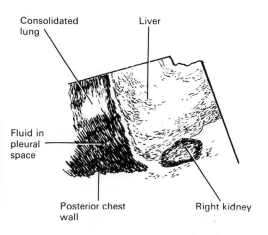

Consolidated
lung

Liver

Fluid in
pleural
space

Posterior chest
wall

Right kidney

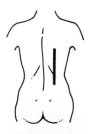

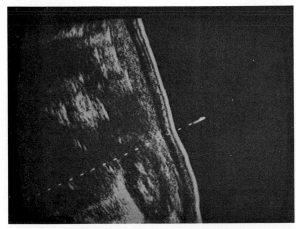

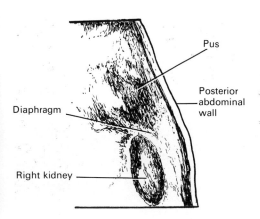

Pus

Posterior
abdominal
wall

Diaphragm

Right kidney

14.3 Pericardial cyst

A 55-year-old white male presented with cough, intermittent low grade fever, and weight loss. Despite antibiotic therapy, persistent opacities were noted on the PA (A) and lateral (B) chest radiographs and the presence of a tumor was suspected clinically. Radiologically, there were some features suggesting the presence of a pericardial cyst; but, because of its irregularity on the lateral tomogram, the possibility of tumor was raised. He was referred for ultrasound examination.

A transverse ultrasonogram of the thorax (C) shows an echo-free area (arrowed) immediately to the right of the heart. An A-scan (D) through this area confirms that this is a cystic lesion. All tests, including bronchoscopy and cytology, were negative for tumor and the patient improved clinically and the infiltrates disappeared. An old chest film was finally traced showing the previous cardiophrenic lesion unchanged, thus confirming its benign nature and the fact that it most likely represented a pericardial cyst. (By kind permission of Dr. Bruce Simonds.)

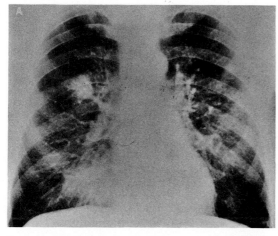

A

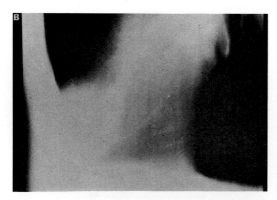

B

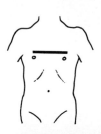

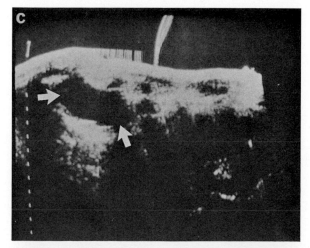

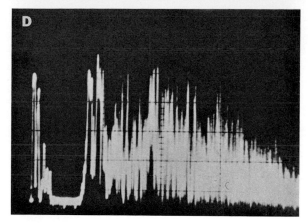

14.4 Fibrous mesothelioma

A 45-year-old female was admitted for diagnostic curettage for postmenopausal bleeding. A preoperative chest X-ray reveals a huge opacity filling the left side of the chest and displacing the heart toward the right. She was referred for ultrasonic evaluation of the heart.

A longitudinal ultrasonogram 7 cm to the right of the midline (upper figure) shows the right lobe of the liver, the gallbladder, and the right kidney, with the heart immediately above the right hemidiaphragm. This confirmed the massive displacement of the heart.

A transverse scan of the left thorax (lower figure) shows a solid, well-circumscribed mass 14 cm in diameter returning irregular internal echoes. This was confirmed at thoracotomy and the histology proved it to be a fibrous mesothelioma.

These case histories demonstrate how ultrasound may be used to differentiate between solid and cystic masses within the thorax and, in particular, between pericardial cysts and solid masses arising in the thorax. (By kind permission of Mrs. Patricia Donnelly and Dr. Murray Rosenberg, Park City Hospital, Bridgeport, Connecticut.)

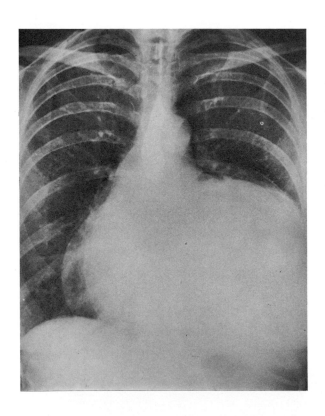

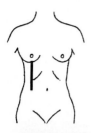

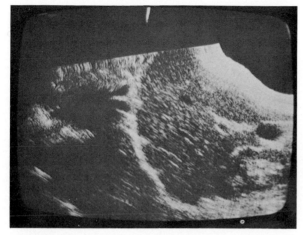

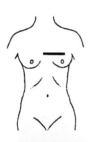

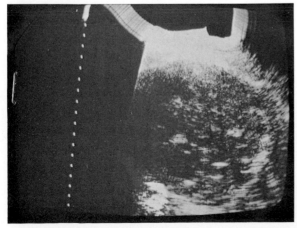